FOOD VALUES

Carbohydrates

D0201418

OTHER BOOKS IN THE FOOD VALUES SERIES

Food Values: Calcium

Food Values: Cholesterol and Fats

FOOD VALUES

Carbohydrates

Leah Wallach

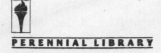

PERENNIAL LIBRARY

Harper & Row, Publishers, New York
Cambridge, Philadelphia, San Francisco
London, Mexico City, São Paulo, Singapore, Sydney

FIRST EDITION

Designed by Alma Orenstein

Library of Congress Cataloging-in-Publication Data

Wallach, Leah, 1947–
     Food values—carbohydrates.

     1. Food—Carbohydrate content—Tables.   2. Carbohydrates
in the body.   I. Title.
TX553.C28W35   1989   641.1′3   88-45623
ISBN 0-06-096220-8

89 90 91 92 93 AG/BC 10 9 8 7 6 5 4 3 2 1

Contents

Acknowledgments

I'd like to thank Laura Hickey, Shawn Connor, and Tim Bishop, who assisted me in the rather tedious task of entering data, and Alex Cantor, who typed and helped organize my correspondence with the food processors. I'd like also to acknowledge Helene A. Guthrie, whom I have never met but whose textbook, *Introductory Nutrition*, proved a most useful reference during the early stages of this project.

I'm especially grateful to Dr. Martin Lipkin of Memorial Sloan-Kettering Cancer Center and Dr. Dennis Ponton, chairman of the Nutrition and Food Science Department, Buffalo State College, who allowed me to consult with them in the course of preparing this book.

Introduction

Everything living runs on sunlight, captured by plants in molecules of carbohydrates. Plants store the radiant energy of light by combining it with water (H_2O) from the soil and carbon (C) from the carbon dioxide in the air to form sugars (simple carbohydrates), starches, and fibers (complex carbohydrates). These molecules supply both plants and animals with the calories they need to grow and move and carry on all the processes of life.

Sugars

There are two basic types of sugars: monosaccharides and disaccharides. Monosaccharides consist of a ring of six carbon atoms and six water molecules. The most important monosaccharides are glucose, also called dextrose and blood sugar; fructose, also called fruit sugar; and galactose.

Glucose, found naturally in fruit, vegetables, and honey, is the principal source of energy for all the organs of the body and the sole source of energy for the brain. It is also the form in which carbohydrate is carried by the blood to the different tissues. All the sugars and starches we eat are broken down in the intestine into glucose, fructose, or galactose. These monosaccharides pass directly through the intestinal wall and are carried to the liver, where they are converted to glucose, which is circulated throughout the body in the blood.

Levels of glucose in the blood go up right after a meal as carbohydrates are digested, then go down as various cells, with the help of insulin, take the glucose they need

om the bloodstream. The levels of glucose in the blood
of a healthy person remain within a certain range, however.
Increased insulin production keeps blood glucose levels
from going too high. When levels fall too low, glucose is
produced from stores of protein and fat.

Fructose occurs naturally in fruit and honey. It can be
absorbed by body cells without the help of insulin, but it
remains in the blood only until it reaches the liver, where
it is converted to glucose. Galactose is formed in the intestine from a more complex sugar in milk; it converts to
glucose when absorbed.

Disaccharides are sugars that consist of a ring of glucose
combined with a second ring of glucose, galactose, or fructose. Disaccharides are broken apart in the intestine to form
monosaccharides.

Sucrose, the most common disaccharide in our diet, is
a combination of glucose and fructose. It occurs naturally
in plants. White sugar, which is refined from sugar cane
and sugar beets, is pure sucrose. Molasses, the syrup that
is drained off when white sugar is processed, is 97% sucrose. Lactose is a combination of glucose and galactose
and is found exclusively in milk and milk products. Maltose,
which consists of two glucose units, is found only in ger-
minating grains. Beer is made by fermenting maltose.

These and other sugars are used to flavor many processed foods. To see if sweeteners have been added to a
product, look for any of these names on the ingredient list:

white sugar	lactose
brown sugar	mannitol
sucrose	honey
glucose	corn syrup
dextrose	molasses
sorbitol	maple syrup
fructose	xylose
maltose	

Starches

Starches are complex carbohydrates called polysacchar-
ides. They are composed of rings of the sugar glucose

linked together in long chains. The flavor, solubility, and thickening power of different starches depend on the number and arrangement of glucose molecules. Starches, like sugars, are broken down into glucose units in the digestive system to make their energy available to our bodies.

The human body stores some carbohydrate, enough for about half a day's energy, in the form of the polysaccharide glycogen. Plants can store carbohydrate energy in the form of sugar, starch, or both. The carbohydrate content of potatoes, grains, mature peas, corn, and unripe fruit, for example, is mostly starch. Ripe fruit, sugar beets, and young peas and corn have a high sugar content—and taste sweet.

Fibers

There are several different kinds of fibers. Most, like starches, are complex carbohydrates, but the human digestive system can't break down the links between the glucose molecules that make up these fibers. Since the fibers can't be digested, they don't supply us with energy. They are nonetheless a valuable part of the diet. They add bulk to the stool, speed the passage of fecal matter through the digestive tract, and may affect the functioning of the microorganisms that naturally inhabit our intestines. There is some evidence that groups of people whose diets are high in fiber have a lower incidence of diverticulitis and cancer of the colon. There is also evidence suggesting that increased intake of certain fibers can lower blood cholesterol levels. (The reader should note, however, that very high intakes of fiber can be too much of a good thing. High fiber consumption can cause irritable bowel syndrome and reduce the absorption of essential minerals.)

Whole grain breads, cereals, and pastas; fruit and vegetables, especially those with edible seeds, stems, and skin; dry beans, peas, nuts, and seeds are all good sources of fiber.

Alcohol

Alcohol is produced by fermenting glucose in sugar, fruits, and grains. Most of the alcohol we consume is used by our bodies as a source of energy.

All the calories in hard liquors like whiskey, gin, and vodka come from alcohol. Only about half the carbohydrates in beer are fermented into alcohol, however, and beer also retains some of the nutrients that were in the grain from which it was made. Wine contributes smaller amounts of carbohydrates and nutrients.

The total amount of alcohol in 12 ounces of beer, 4 ounces of wine, and an ounce-and-a-half shot of distilled hard liquor is about the same. A person who enjoys a two-white-wine lunch is drinking as much alcohol as a person who has a two-bourbon lunch.

Carbohydrates in Our Diet

Carbohydrates, protein, fat, and water are the basic nutrients that make up the bulk of our diet. We also need tiny amounts of vitamins and minerals, which facilitate chemical reactions in the body, maintain the balance of body fluids, and are used as components of some cells and cell products.

Most Americans now get 40% to 45% of their food energy—calories—directly from carbohydrates of all kinds. From 12% to 24% of our daily caloric intake—different sources give different values—comes from sugars alone.

The health-conscious have always tried to avoid sugary desserts, which nutritionists agree is a good idea, but nutritionists do not think it's a good idea to reduce total carbohydrate consumption, which many dieters have also tried to do. For years, people watching their weight have ignored the potatoes and rejected the charms of big bowls of spaghetti. Beef, chicken, or fish eaten with a green salad and no starch was considered an admirable dinner. That's a mistake, according to public health officials. The U.S. Department of Agriculture now recommends that we increase our intake of carbohydrates to about 55% of our total calories and reduce proportionately our consumption of fat. They also recommend decreasing the carbohydrate calories supplied by sugars to about 10% of total calories, through cutting back consumption of processed foods and beverages prepared with added sweeteners.

Sugar and Health

Sugar has gotten terrible press: some books and article give the impression that it's a low-grade poison. It's not Inside our body, it is sugar, in the form of glucose, that provides us with the energy we need to think, play, and work. The sugar in foods makes them taste good. And sugar is not guilty of many of the evil effects that have been attributed to it.

Sugar does not make people fat; excess calories make people fat. People gain weight when their diets contain more food energy than they use. Sugar, starch, and protein all contain about 4 calories per gram. Fat contains 9 calories per gram. Cutting down on fat consumption is a more efficient way to cut calories than cutting back on sugar.

Sugar does not cause diabetes. Diabetics have elevated blood sugar (hyperglycemia), not because they eat more sugar than other people, but because their pancreas does not produce enough insulin to help cells remove glucose from the bloodstream.

Some diabetics can regulate their condition by regulating the amount of carbohydrate in their diet, so that glucose is not released into their bloodstream rapidly. These patients used to be advised specifically to reduce sugar consumption and to replace sugars with starches. It was believed that simple sugars would raise blood sugar levels faster than starches, which must be broken down into sugar units. This sounds reasonable, but when researchers began to measure the effects of different foods on blood sugar levels and compared them with the effects of eating pure glucose, they found that some starches raise the level of sugar in the blood faster than some sugars.

People who produce too much insulin have a condition called spontaneous hypoglycemia. Their blood sugar levels are chronically low. Most people occasionally experience a mild, very transient form of hypoglycemia, which is related to eating. If a person waits too long between meals, the cells begin to deplete the sugar in the blood faster than the liver can restore it, and blood sugar levels drop for a little while. Reactive hypoglycemia can also follow consumption of a high-carbohydrate meal. The sudden increase in blood

ar as the meal is digested can overstimulate the pan-
as so that it temporarily produces too much insulin.

There have been numerous reports linking hyperactivity
n children to sugar consumption, but scientific studies thus
far have not confirmed the link. There is some preliminary
evidence that diets high in both fructose and fat may increase the risk of coronary heart disease, but considerably
more research is needed to see if this relationship is real
and significant.

There is only one health problem that has clearly been
linked to sugar consumption: dental cavities. Carbohydrates
feed bacteria that live in the mouth and cause tooth decay.
Sticky sugary foods like caramels and dried apricots do the
most damage. One of the reasons why nutritionists recommend that we reduce our intake of sugar is to reduce
the incidence of tooth decay. (Cleaning one's teeth after
eating a sticky sweet helps too.)

The other reason why nutritionists recommend reduced
intake of added sweeteners is that they provide virtually no
vitamins, minerals, or fiber. Honey and brown sugar have
a reputation for being nutritious, but it's unfounded. Nutritionists recommend that we get our carbohydrate calories
from complex carbohydrates and naturally sweet foods,
rather than from added sweeteners, because that way we
get more nutrition for our food energy.

Carbohydrates and Mood

Not only have scientific studies failed to find any connec-
tion between sugar consumption and hyperactivity, but another line of research suggests that meals rich in carbohydrates—sugars or starches—may make people *less*
agitated. Researchers believe that carbohydrate consumption may affect mood, not by changing blood sugar levels,
but indirectly, by increasing levels of the neurotransmitter
serotonin in the brain. Neurotransmitters, as their name im-
plies, are chemicals that help transmit messages from one
nerve cell to another.

The strongest evidence for the hypothesis that carbohydrate consumption increases serotonin production comes
from experiments done on rats. The results of studies done

on people have been inconsistent. What's more, the of elevating levels of different neurotransmitters are no understood and may depend on their interaction with o neurotransmitters and on the situation. High levels of s otonin, for example, have been associated with feelings o relaxation, confidence, and focus—and also with drowsiness, sluggishness, and lassitude. More work clearly needs to be done before attempting to manipulate mood by changing diet.

Carbohydrates, Fat, and Calories

Plants contain fat and protein as well as carbohydrates. A few plant foods—nuts, for example—have a high fat content, but fruit and vegetables generally contain much less fat than animal foods. We like the taste of fat, however, and habitually add fat to low-fat vegetable foods: we put butter or margarine on bread and vegetables, sauté meats, cover pasta in cheese and cream sauces, pour oil dressings over salad. Increasing the percentage of calories in our diet that comes from carbohydrates while reducing the percentage that comes from fats means making more moderate use of butter and oils in cooking, reducing the quantities of butter, margarine, dressings, and mayonnaise used as condiments, and using heavy sauces less frequently.

Plants do not contain cholesterol, but they do contain saturated fats, which raise the level of cholesterol in the blood more than dietary cholesterol does. Most of the oils extracted from fruit and vegetables are lower in saturated fat than animal fats, but the most saturated fat in our diet, coconut oil, comes from a plant.

Those concerned about weight control would do best to concentrate on reducing fat intake. Dieters can also reduce carbohydrate intake to lower their total calorie consumption—but they shouldn't try to eliminate carbohydrates altogether. Without sufficient carbohydrate intake, the process of converting fat to fuel is disrupted, and by-products of the incomplete fat metabolism called ketones build up in the body, causing dehydration and loss of energy. A healthy weight-control diet should include a *minimum* of 100 grams of carbohydrates—about 400 calories' worth.

How to Use This Book

Food Values: Carbohydrates provides the number of grams of carbohydrates and the total number of calories in thousands of foods.

The foods are divided into forty-eight categories covering all the things we eat and drink. As you flip through the pages of this book you'll quickly see where various foods are located. If you can't find a food in the category where you think it belongs, check the head note at the beginning of the category or refer to the table of contents. When products could be classified in more than one category, we have tried to include a "see also" reference.

Each category begins with an alphabetical listing of generic food items, with fresh products listed before processed foods; for instance, you'll find fresh peaches before canned peaches. Following the generic foods are all brand-name products alphabetized by the name that is most easily recognized, either the name of the manufacturing company, of the product line, or of the product itself. For instance, Campbell's soups are listed under Campbell, the company name, while Ortega sauces are listed under Ortega, the product line name, rather than under the manufacturer, Nabisco, and Kit Kat candy bar is listed under Kit Kat, because the product name is better known than the fact that it is a Hershey product. Under each brand name, specific products are generally listed alphabetically; Aunt Jemima French toast, for example, precedes Aunt Jemima pancakes. We found, however, as most alphabetizers do, that some items could be listed in more than one way; we had to make choices. Diet Slice soft drink immediately follows Slice in

everage listings, for instance, even though it begins
d, while split peas are under *s* not *p*. If you don't find
od under the first letter of the first word of its name,
looking for it under the first letter of another word in
he name. The cross-references should help here too.

Be sure to look for foods in the form in which you eat
them: the way foods are prepared and measured changes
their nutrient values. A cup of canned cling peaches with
syrup contains fewer peaches and more sugar syrup than a
cup of drained cling peaches. A dry soup mix prepared with
skim milk will have fewer calories than the same mix prepared with half and half.

We've used the portion sizes that Americans use—cups,
ounces, or serving units—and when available, we've used
two kinds of measures; for example, "3 cookies = 1 oz."
Serving units are the easiest portions to measure: it's easier
to count cookies than to weigh them. However, you can only
compare serving units of the same weight. For example, if
a package of Brand X frozen lasagna weighs 10 ounces,
and a package of Brand Y frozen lasagna weighs 18 ounces,
the calorie and carbohydrate figures will be higher for Brand
Y than for Brand X, because the portion size is bigger. But
Brand Y might contain fewer carbohydrates or calories per
ounce than Brand X. To compare two products of different
sizes, divide the values for each product by the number of
ounces it contains, and then compare the values for 1
ounce.

Please note the difference between weight measures and
volume measures. Measuring cups measure fluid ounces.
An ounce of water by weight fills a measuring cup to the
1-ounce line. But volume and weight are very different kinds
of measures for solid foods. An ounce of unpopped popcorn, which is dense, wouldn't fill a measuring cup, for
example, but an ounce of popped popcorn, which is airy,
would fill more than one. In this book, portions for solid
food given in ounces refer to weight. Fluid ounces (fl oz),
cups (c), teaspoons (t), and tablespoons (T) refer to volume
measurements. Since we don't ordinarily weigh our food,
we've given volume and weight measurements when both
are available and useful. For example, we've indicated how
much of a measuring cup would be filled by an ounce of
a given cold cereal when this information was available.

All the values given here are approximations. No two apples, chicken breasts, or rolls are exactly alike. Data represent averages for several samples.

Figures provided by different sources may not be exactly comparable. The U.S. Department of Agriculture (USDA) and various manufacturers may use different analytical procedures to analyze nutrient content and may round off the data in different ways. In the USDA *Composition of Food* series, our source of information about generic and fresh food, values are given to hundredths or thousandths. We rounded off the figures to the nearest whole unit. For example, we list 68.4 calories as 68 calories and 68.5 calories as 69 calories. When an item contained less than .5 calorie or less than .5 gram of carbohydrate, we listed the value as a "trace" (tr) (1 gram equals .035 ounce).

Many manufacturers use a simpler rounding-off system for calories, approved by the Food and Drug Administration, which regulates food labels. Calories between 0 and 20 may be given in increments of 2; between 20 and 50 in increments of 5; and above 50 in increments of 5 or 10. This means that there's no point in counting single calories when comparing products; a product listed as containing 197 calories, another listed as containing 195 calories, and a third listed as containing 200 calories may actually contain the same amount of food energy. For most practical purposes, these small differences don't matter. If you need about 2,000 calories a day, it doesn't matter if you get 2,005 one day and 1,991 the next.

This book contains the best and most complete information now available. When information about the content of a particular nutrient in a food was not available or has not been determined, we put a question mark in the appropriate column. Since food manufacturers constantly change recipes and product sizes and develop new products, some of the data contained here may quickly become outdated.

Calculating the Number of Grams of Carbohydrate in Your Diet

To find the amount of carbohydrate in your diet, keep a complete record of everything you eat and drink (including small snacks) for three days, one of which should be a weekend day. Right after you finish a meal or snack, write down what you ate, how it was prepared, and the portion by volume (cups, teaspoons), weight (pounds, ounces), or units (1 piece of fruit, 1 English muffin), or all three if you can. At home, measure your food. For example, instead of just pouring milk from the carton over your cereal, pour it into a measuring cup first to see how much you use. Use tablespoons to measure the milk you pour into your tea or coffee. If you measure your foods at home, you'll begin to get a feeling for different sizes and be able to estimate portions better when you eat out. You will probably find that the portion sizes used in the book are on the small side. For many adult Americans, for example, a typical portion of spaghetti is 2 cups—not the 1 cup listed as a portion here.

At the end of three days, look up the carbohydrate and calorie values for every food on your list. Add them up and divide by three to get your average daily intake of each.

Calculating the Percentage of Calories Supplied by Carbohydrate in Your Diet

A gram of carbohydrate contains about 4 calories. To find the number of calories supplied by carbohydrates in a given food, multiply the number of grams of carbohydrate in the food by 4. To find the percentage of calories supplied by carbohydrate, divide the number of calories supplied by carbohydrate by the total number of calories. For example, a Sunshine fig bar contains 11 grams of carbohydrate. Multiplying 11 grams of carbohydrate by 4 calories gives 44 calories. The total number of calories in the cookie is 45. Dividing 44 by 45 tells us that about 98% of the calories in the cookie come from carbohydrate.

Use the same procedure to calculate the percentage of calories supplied by carbohydrates in a given meal or a whole day: add together the grams of carbohydrate in all the foods and beverages you consume and multiply by 4 to get the calories supplied by carbohydrate. Add together the total calories in all foods and beverages. The total carbohydrate calories divided by the total calories gives you the

fraction or percentage of total calories supplied by carbo
hydrate.

This procedure is approximate only. The amount of energy the body gets from nutrients varies slightly from food
to food and meal to meal. In addition, the carbohydrate
values may include some fibers, which are not digested and
yield no energy at all; this means that the figure you get for
carbohydrate calories using the 1-gram-of-carbohydrate-
equals-4-calories system may be on the high side for high-
fiber foods. The method is accurate enough for all practical
purposes, however, and is used by many professional nutritionists for meal planning.

Sources

1. *Food Values of Portions Commonly Used, 14th Edition*, Jean A. T. Pennington and Helen Nichols Church, Harper & Row, 1985.
2. *Nutritive Value of Foods*, U.S. Department of Agriculture, Nutrition Information Service, Home and Garden Bulletin #72, revised 1981.
3. *Composition of Food Series*, U.S. Department of Agriculture, Science and Education Administration:

   8-1 *Dairy and Egg Products*, revised November 1976.
   8-3 *Baby Foods*, revised December 1978.
   8-4 *Fats and Oils*, revised June 1979.
   8-5 *Poultry Products*, revised August 1979.
   8-6 *Soups, Sauces and Gravies*, revised February 1980.
   8-7 *Sausages and Luncheon Meats*, revised September 1980.
   8-8 *Breakfast Cereals*, revised July 1982.
   8-9 *Fruits and Fruit Juices*, revised August 1982.
   8-10 *Pork Products*, revised August 1983.
   8-11 *Vegetables and Vegetable Products*, revised August 1984.
   8-12 *Nut and Seed Products*, revised September 1984.
   8-13 *Beef Products*, revised August 1986.
   8-14 *Beverages*, revised May 1986.
   8-15 *Finfish and Shellfish Products*, revised September 1987.
   8-16 *Legumes and Legume Products*, revised December 1986.

Information about brand-name products was supplied by the food processing companies themselves or taken from the above sources.

Abbreviations

c	=	cup
cal	=	calories
diam	=	diameter
g	=	grams
lb	=	pounds
mg	=	milligrams
oz	=	ounces
pkg	=	package
pkt	=	packet
T	=	tablespoon
t	=	teaspoon
tr	=	trace
w/	=	with
w/out	=	without
?	=	not available, or not known at this time
<	=	less than
≤	=	less than or equal to

FOOD VALUES
Carbohydrates

	Portion	Carbohydrates (g)	Total Calories

◻ ALCOHOLIC BEVERAGES
See BEVERAGES

◻ BABY FOOD *See* INFANT & TODDLER FOODS

◻ BAKING INGREDIENTS

	Portion	Carbohydrates (g)	Total Calories
baking powder, all types	1 t	1	5
baking soda	1 t	0	0
candied fruit			
apricot	1 medium	26	101
cherry	3 large	13	51
maraschino cherry	2 medium	5	19
citron	1 oz	23	89
fig	1 piece	22	90
ginger root	1 oz	24	95
peel of grapefruit/lemon/ orange	1 oz	23	89
pear	1 oz	21	85
pineapple	1 slice	30	120
cornmeal *See* FLOURS & CORNMEALS			
cornstarch *See* FLOURS & CORNMEALS			
flour *See* FLOURS & CORNMEALS			
pastry puff dough	1 oz	8	129
patty shell	2½ oz	15	240
piecrust			
crumb	5.8 oz	64	866
from mix w/vegetable shortening	for 2-crust 9″ pie	141	1,485
from sticks	⅛ double crust = 2 oz	27	290
frozen	1/16 crust = 1 oz	14	130
graham cracker	4.8 oz	18	159
homemade, w/vegetable shortening	for 9″ pie	79	900
yeast			
baker's, dry, active	1 pkg	3	20
brewer's, dry	1 T	3	25
torula	1 T	4	28

	Portion	Carbohydrates (g)	Total Calories
BRAND NAME			
Baker's			
COCONUT			
Angel Flake, bag	⅓ c	10	120
CHOCOLATE			
German's sweet chocolate	1 oz	17	140
semisweet chocolate	1 oz	17	140
semisweet chocolate–flavored chips	¼ c	31	190
semisweet real chocolate chips	¼ c	28	200
unsweetened chocolate	1 oz	9	140
Davis			
baking powder	1 t	2	8
Hershey			
milk chocolate chips	1 oz	18	150
semisweet chocolate chips, regular & miniature	¼ c or 1½ oz	26	220
unsweetened baking chocolate	1 oz	7	190
Nabisco			
graham cracker crumbs	2 T	11	60
Reese's			
peanut butter–flavored chips	¼ c or 1½ oz	19	230
Sunshine			
graham cracker crumbs	1 c	95	550

☐ BAKING MIXES

all-purpose biscuit/pancake mix	½ c	38	240

cakes & pastries, prepared from mix *See* DESSERTS: CAKES, PASTRIES, & PIES
pancakes, prepared from mix *See* BREAKFAST FOODS, PREPARED
pie fillings, prepared from mix *See* DESSERTS: CUSTARDS, GELATINS, PUDDINGS, & PIE FILLINGS
waffles, prepared from mix *See* BREAKFAST FOODS, PREPARED

■ BRAND NAME

Arrowhead Mills			
biscuit mix	2 oz	19	100
bran muffin mix	2 muffins	43	270
corn bread mix	1 oz	19	100

	Portion	Carbohydrates (g)	Total Calories
Aunt Jemima			
Easy Mix coffee cake	1.3 oz	29	162
Easy Mix corn bread	1.7 oz	34	205
Dromedary			
corn bread, prepared	2"×2" piece	20	130
corn muffin, prepared	1 muffin	20	120
gingerbread, prepared	2"×2" piece	19	100
pound cake, prepared	½" slice	21	150
Fearn			
BAKING MIXES			
brown rice	½ c	41	215
rice	½ c	54	260
whole-wheat	½ c	45	210
BREAD & MUFFIN MIXES			
bran muffin	1½ oz	27	110
corn bread	⅓ c dry	30	160
CAKE MIXES			
banana	⅓ c dry	26	130
carob	⅓ c dry	25	120
carrot	⅓ c dry	26	140
spice	⅓ c dry	24	140
Flako			
corn muffin mix	1 oz	20	116
pie crust mix	1.7 oz	25	244
popover mix	1 oz	20	102
Jell-O			
cheesecake, prepared w/whole milk	⅛ of 8" cake	36	280
chocolate mousse pie, prepared w/whole milk	⅛ pie	28	250
coconut cream pie, prepared w/whole milk	⅛ pie	27	260
Pillsbury			
All Ready pie crust	⅛ of 2-crust pie	24	240
Royal			
chocolate mint pie mix	⅛ pie	25	260
chocolate mousse pie mix	⅛ pie	27	230
lemon meringue pie mix	⅛ pie	50	310
lite cheese cake mix	⅛ pie	23	210
Real cheese cake mix	⅛ pie	31	280

❑ **BEANS** *See* LEGUMES
& LEGUME PRODUCTS

	Portion	Carbohydrates (g)	Total Calories

❑ BEEF, FRESH & CURED
See also PROCESSED MEAT & POULTRY PRODUCTS

Beef, Fresh

RETAIL CUTS

Retail cuts of fresh muscle meat (steaks, roasts, ground meat) contain virtually no carbohydrates.

VARIETY MEATS

	Portion	Carbohydrates (g)	Total Calories
brains			
pan-fried	3 oz cooked	0	167
simmered	3 oz cooked	0	136
heart, simmered	3 oz cooked	tr	148
kidneys, simmered	3 oz cooked	1	122
liver			
braised	3 oz cooked	3	137
pan-fried	3 oz cooked	7	184
lungs, braised	3 oz cooked	0	102
suet, raw	1 oz	0	242
tongue, simmered	3 oz cooked	tr	241
tripe, raw	1 oz	0	28
	4 oz	0	111

Beef, Cured

	Portion	Carbohydrates (g)	Total Calories
breakfast strips, cooked	3 (15 per 12 oz pkg)	tr	153
	6 oz	2	764
corned beef brisket, braised	3 oz cooked	tr	213
	1 lb raw	2	802

▪ BRAND NAME

Oscar Mayer

	Portion	Carbohydrates (g)	Total Calories
breakfast strips, cooked	1 (15 per 12 oz pkg)	tr	46

❑ BEVERAGES
See also FAST FOODS; MILK, MILK SUBSTITUTES, & MILK PRODUCTS

Beverages, Alcoholic

BEER & ALE

	Portion	Carbohydrates (g)	Total Calories
ale, mild	8 fl oz	80	98

	Portion	Carbohydrates (g)	Total Calories
beer			
regular (4½% alcohol by volume)	12 fl oz	13	146
light (alcohol & carbohydrate content of light beer vary)	12 fl oz	5	100

COCKTAILS & MIXED DRINKS

	Portion	Carbohydrates (g)	Total Calories
Bloody Mary	5 fl oz	5	116
bourbon & soda	4 fl oz	0	105
daiquiri, canned	6.8 fl oz	?	?
daiquiri cocktail	2 fl oz	4	111
eggnog *See* Flavored Milk Beverages, *below*			
gin & tonic	7½ fl oz	16	171
Gin Rickey	4 fl oz	1	150
manhattan	2 fl oz	2	128
martini	2½ fl oz	tr	156
piña colada, canned	6.8 fl oz	61	525
piña colada cocktail	4½ fl oz	40	262
planter's punch	3½ fl oz	8	175
screwdriver	7 fl oz	18	174
tequila sunrise	5½ fl oz	15	189
Tom Collins	7½ fl oz	3	121
whiskey sour, canned	6.8 fl oz	?	?
whiskey sour cocktail	3 fl oz	5	123
whiskey sour mix			
powder	1 pkt	16	64
prepared w/water & whiskey	1 pkt + 1½ fl oz water + 1½ fl oz whiskey	16	169
bottled (no alcohol)	2 fl oz	14	55
prepared w/whiskey	2 fl oz mix + 1½ fl oz whiskey	14	158

CORDIALS & LIQUEURS

	Portion	Carbohydrates (g)	Total Calories
54 proof (22.1% alcohol by weight)	1 fl oz	12	97
coffee liqueur (53 proof)	1½ fl oz	24	174
coffee w/cream liqueur (34 proof)	1½ fl oz	10	154
crème de menthe liqueur (72 proof)	1½ fl oz	21	186

DISTILLED SPIRITS

	Portion	Carbohydrates (g)	Total Calories
all (gin, rum, vodka, whiskey)			
100 proof	1 fl oz	0	82
	1½ fl oz	0	124
94 proof	1 fl oz	0	76
	1½ fl oz	0	116
gin, 90 proof	1½ fl oz	0	110

	Portion	Carbohydrates (g)	Total Calories
rum, 80 proof	1½ fl oz	0	97
vodka, 80 proof	1½ fl oz	0	97
whiskey, 86 proof	1½ fl oz	tr	105

WINES

	Portion	Carbohydrates (g)	Total Calories
champagne	4 fl oz	3	84
dessert wine, sweet, 18.8% alcohol by volume	1 fl oz	4	46
muscatel or port	3½ fl oz	14	158
sauterne	3½ fl oz	4	84
sherry	2 fl oz	5	84
table wine, 11½% alcohol by volume			
all	1 fl oz	tr	21
	3½ fl oz	1	72
red	1 fl oz	1	21
	3½ fl oz	2	74
rosé	1 fl oz	tr	21
	3½ fl oz	2	73
white	1 fl oz	tr	20
	3½ fl oz	1	70
vermouth, dry, French	3½ fl oz	1	105

Beverages, Carbonated

	Portion	Carbohydrates (g)	Total Calories
bitter lemon	12 fl oz	47	192
club soda	12 fl oz	0	0
cola	12 fl oz	39	151
low-cal, aspartame-sweetened	12 fl oz	tr	2
low-cal, sodium-saccharin-sweetened	12 fl oz	0	2
cream soda	12 fl oz	49	191
diet soda, all flavors	12 fl oz	tr	0
ginger ale	12 fl oz	32	124
grape soda	12 fl oz	42	161
lemon-lime soda	12 fl oz	38	149
orange soda	12 fl oz	46	177
peach soda	12 fl oz	46	184
quinine water	4 fl oz	10	37
root beer	12 fl oz	39	152
strawberry soda	12 fl oz	44	174
tonic water	12 fl oz	32	125

Coffee & Coffee Substitutes

	Portion	Carbohydrates (g)	Total Calories
coffee, brewed	6 fl oz	1	4
coffee, instant, regular or decaffeinated, powder, prepared w/water	6 fl oz water + 1 rounded t powder	1	4

	Portion	Carbohydrates (g)	Total Calories
coffee substitute, cereal grain beverage, powder			
prepared w/water	6 fl oz water + 1 t powder	2	9
prepared w/whole milk	6 fl oz milk + 1 t powder	10	121

Flavored Milk Beverages

	Portion	Carbohydrates (g)	Total Calories
carob-flavored mix			
powder	3 t	11	45
powder, prepared w/whole milk	1 c milk + 3 t powder	23	195
chocolate dairy drink, reduced-calorie, aspartame-sweetened, powder, prepared w/ water	½ c water + 3 ice cubes + ¾ oz pkt	11	64
chocolate-flavored mix			
powder	2–3 heaping t	20	75
powder, prepared w/whole milk	1 c milk + 2–3 heaping t powder	31	226
chocolate milk			
whole	1 c	26	208
low-fat, 2%	1 c	26	179
low-fat, 1%	1 c	26	158
chocolate syrup			
w/added nutrients	1 T	12	46
prepared w/whole milk	1 c milk + 1 T syrup	24	196
w/out added nutrients	1 fl oz	22	82
prepared w/whole milk	1 c milk + 2 T syrup	34	232
cocoa, homemade, w/whole milk	6 fl oz	19	164
	1 c	26	218
cocoa mix			
reduced-calorie, aspartame-sweetened, powder, prepared w/water	6 fl oz water + .53 oz pkt	9	48
w/added nutrients	6 fl oz water + 1 pkt	24	120
w/out added nutrients	6 fl oz water + 3–4 heaping t powder	23	103
eggnog, dairy	1 c	34	342
eggnog-flavored mix, powder, prepared w/whole milk	1 c milk + 2 heaping t powder	39	260
malt beverage	12 fl oz	5	32

	Portion	Carbohydrates (g)	Total Calories
malted milk–flavored mix, chocolate			
w/added nutrients			
powder	¾ oz or 4–5 heaping t	18	75
powder, prepared w/whole milk	1 c milk + 4–5 heaping t powder	29	225
w/out added nutrients			
powder	¾ oz or 3 heaping t	18	79
powder, prepared w/whole milk	1 c milk + 3 heaping t powder	30	229
malted milk–flavored mix, natural			
w/added nutrients			
powder	¾ oz or 4–5 heaping t	17	80
powder, prepared w/whole milk	1 c milk + 4–5 heaping t powder	28	230
w/out added nutrients			
powder	¾ oz or 3 heaping t	16	87
powder, prepared w/whole milk	1 c milk + 3 heaping t powder	27	237
shake, thick			
chocolate	10 oz	60	335
vanilla	10 oz	50	315
strawberry-flavored mix, powder, prepared w/whole milk	1 c milk + 2–3 heaping t powder	33	234

Fruit & Vegetable Juices

	Portion	Carbohydrates (g)	Total Calories
acerola	1 c	12	51
apple			
canned or bottled	1 c	29	116
from frozen concentrate	1 c	28	111
apricot, canned	1 c	36	141
carrot, canned	½ c	11	49
cranberry, bottled	1 c	38	147
grape			
canned	1 c	38	155
from frozen concentrate, sweetened	1 c	32	128
grapefruit			
fresh	1 c	23	96

	Portion	Carbohydrates (g)	C
canned			
sweetened	1 c	28	11
unsweetened	1 c	22	93
from frozen concentrate	1 c	24	102
lemon			
fresh	1 T	1	4
canned or bottled	1 T	1	3
frozen, single strength	1 T	1	3
lime			
fresh	1 T	1	4
canned or bottled	1 T	1	3
orange			
fresh	1 c	26	111
canned	1 c	25	104
from frozen concentrate	1 c	27	112
frozen concentrate, undiluted	6 fl oz	81	339
orange-grapefruit, canned	1 c	25	107
papaya, canned	1 c	36	142
passion fruit			
purple	1 c	34	126
yellow	1 c	36	149
peach, canned	1 c	35	134
pear, canned	1 c	39	149
pineapple			
canned	1 c	34	139
from frozen concentrate	1 c	32	129
prune, canned	1 c	45	181
tangerine			
fresh	1 c	25	106
canned, sweetened	1 c	30	125
from frozen concentrate, sweetened	1 c	27	110
tomato, canned	6 fl oz	8	32
w/beef broth	5½ fl oz	14	61
w/clam juice	5½ fl oz	18	77
vegetable, canned	6 fl oz	8	34

Fruit Juice Drinks (10–50% Fruit Juice), Juice Ades, & Juice-flavored Drinks & Powders

apple juice drink, canned	6 fl oz	23	92
cherry juice drink, canned	6 fl oz	23	93
citrus fruit drink, canned	6 fl oz	23	93
citrus fruit juice drink, from frozen concentrate	1 c	28	114
cranberry-apple juice drink			
bottled	6 fl oz	32	123
canned	6 fl oz	35	135
cranberry-apricot juice drink, bottled	6 fl oz	30	118

	Portion	Carbohydrates (g)	Total Calories
erry-grape juice drink, ottled	6 fl oz	26	103
nberry juice cocktail			
ottled	6 fl oz	27	108
rom frozen concentrate	6 fl oz	26	102
low-cal, calcium-saccharin- & corn-sweetened, bottled	6 fl oz	9	33
fruit juice drink, from mix, average for 9 flavors	6 fl oz	18	70
fruit punch drink			
canned	6 fl oz	22	87
from frozen concentrate	1 c	29	113
fruit punch–flavored drink, powder, prepared w/water	1 c water + 2 rounded T powder	25	97
fruit punch juice drink			
canned	6 fl oz	25	99
from frozen concentrate	1 c	30	123
gelatin drink, orange-flavored, powder	0.6 oz pkt	11	67
grape drink, canned	6 fl oz	22	84
grape juice drink, canned	6 fl oz	24	94
lemonade			
from frozen concentrate	1 c	26	100
powder, prepared w/water	1 c water + 2 T powder	27	102
powder, low-cal, aspartame-sweetened	0.42 oz pkt	10	40
	0.67 oz pkt	16	63
lemonade-flavored drink, powder, prepared w/water	1 c water + 2 T powder	29	113
lemon-lime, from mix	8 fl oz	23	91
limeade, from frozen concentrate	1 c	27	102
orange & apricot juice drink, canned	1 c	32	128
orange drink, canned	6 fl oz	24	94
orange drink, breakfast type, from frozen concentrate (orange juice & orange pulp)	6 fl oz	21	84
orange-flavored drink, breakfast type			
from frozen concentrate w/orange pulp	6 fl oz	23	91
from powder	3 rounded t powder + 6 fl oz water	22	86
orange juice drink, canned	6 fl oz	23	92
orange-pineapple juice drink, canned	6 fl oz	23	94

	Portion	Carbohydrates (g)	Total Calories
peach juice drink, canned	6 fl oz	23	90
pineapple & grapefruit juice drink, canned	1 c	29	117
pineapple & orange juice drink, canned	1 c	29	125
pineapple-orange juice drink, canned	6 fl oz	24	99
strawberry juice drink, canned	6 fl oz	22	89
tangerine juice drink, canned	6 fl oz	23	90
wild berry juice drink, canned	6 fl oz	22	88

Tea

brewed	6 fl oz	tr	2
herb, brewed	6 fl oz	tr	1
iced, canned, sweetened	12 fl oz	37	146
instant, powder			
low-cal, sodium-saccharin-sweetened, lemon-flavored	2 t	1	5
sugar-sweetened, lemon-flavored	3 rounded t	22	87
sweetened	3 t in 8 fl oz water	22	86
unsweetened	1 t	tr	2
unsweetened, lemon-flavored	1 rounded t	1	4

Water

municipal	1 c	0	0

▪ BRAND NAME

Apple & Eve Juices

apple	6 fl oz	19	75
apple cranberry	6 fl oz	19	75
apple grape	6 fl oz	21	83
cranberry-grape	6 fl oz	23	94
raspberry-cranberry	6 fl oz	21	86
vegetable	6 fl oz	7	34

Awake

from frozen concentrate	6 fl oz	22	91

Bright & Early

imitation orange beverage, from carton or frozen concentrate	6 fl oz	12	90

Campbell Juices

apple	6 oz	23	100
appleberry	6 oz	24	100
cherry	6 oz	24	100

	Portion	Carbohydrates (g)	Total Calories
grape	6 oz	23	100
orange	6 oz	22	90
strawberry	6 oz	24	100
tomato	6 oz	8	35
Coca-Cola Soft Drinks			
Classic	6 fl oz	19	72
Coca-Cola	6 fl oz	20	77
Caffeine-Free	6 fl oz	20	77
Diet Coke	6 fl oz	tr	1
Caffeine-Free Diet Coke	6 fl oz	tr	1
cherry	6 fl oz	20	76
diet cherry	6 fl oz	tr	1
Fresca	6 fl oz	tr	2
Max Sports Drink	6 fl oz	5	35
Mello Yello	6 fl oz	22	87
Mr. Pibb	12 fl oz	38	143
Diet Mr. Pibb	12 fl oz	tr	1
Ramblin' Root Beer	6 fl oz	23	88
Sprite	6 fl oz	18	71
Diet Sprite	6 fl oz	2	0
Tab	6 fl oz	tr	tr
Caffeine-Free Tab	6 fl oz	tr	tr
Country Time Drink Mix			
lemonade & pink lemonade			
sugar-sweetened	8 fl oz	20	80
w/NutraSweet	8 fl oz	0	4
lemon-lime, sugar-sweetened	8 fl oz	20	80
Crystal Light Drink Mix			
all flavors except tropical fruit	8 fl oz	0	4
tropical fruit	8 fl oz	1	4
Diet Rite			
soda	12 fl oz	tr	1
Dole Juices			
pineapple	6 oz	25	103
pineapple–pink grapefruit	6 oz	25	101
New pineapple	6 oz	25	100
New pineapple-grapefruit	6 oz	23	90
New pineapple-orange	6 oz	23	100
Dr. Pepper Soft Drinks			
Dr. Pepper	6 fl oz	19	72
Diet Dr. Pepper	6 fl oz	tr	1
Caffeine-Free Pepper Free	6 fl oz	19	72
Diet Pepper Free	6 fl oz	tr	1
Fanta Soft Drinks			
ginger ale	6 fl oz	16	63
grape	6 fl oz	22	86
orange	6 fl oz	23	88
root beer	6 fl oz	20	78

	Portion	Carbohydrates (g)	

Featherweight
hot cocoa, low-cal	6 oz	7	
tomato juice, low-sodium	6 oz	8	3

Five Alive Fruit Drinks
CARTONS
berry citrus	6 fl oz	12	88
citrus	6 fl oz	12	87
tropical citrus	6 fl oz	12	88

FROZEN CONCENTRATE
all flavors except fruit punch	6 fl oz	12	85–87
fruit punch	6 fl oz	23	87

Gatorade
lemon-lime or orange flavor, w/ water	8 fl oz	15	60

Hawaiian Punch
Fruit Juicy Red
regular	6 fl oz	22	90
light	6 fl oz	15	60
grape	6 fl oz	23	90
Island Fruit Cocktail	6 fl oz	22	90
orange	6 fl oz	24	100
tropical fruit	6 fl oz	22	90
Very Berry	6 fl oz	22	90
Wild Fruit	6 fl oz	23	90

Hershey
chocolate-flavored syrup	2 T	17	80
chocolate milk, 2% low-fat	1 c	29	190
cocoa	⅓ c	13	120
instant cocoa	3 T	17	80

Hi-C Fruit Drinks
Double Fruit Cooler	6 fl oz	23	86
Fruit Punch	6 fl oz	23	92
100 Apple	6 fl oz	22	89
100 Grape	6 fl oz	23	94
100 Orange	6 fl oz	23	94

International Coffees
all coffees, sugar-free	6 fl oz	3	25–35
Cafe Amaretto	6 fl oz	7	50
Cafe Français	6 fl oz	6	50
Cafe Irish Creme	6 fl oz	8	60
Cafe Vienna	6 fl oz	10	60
Double Dutch Chocolate	6 fl oz	8	50
Irish Mocha Mint	6 fl oz	8	50
Orange Cappuccino	6 fl oz	10	60
Suisse Mocha	6 fl oz	8	50

	Portion	Carbohydrates (g)	Total Calories
RS			
ntain Berry punch	8.45 fl oz	31	130
abow punch	8.45 fl oz	34	130
opical punch	8.45 fl oz	35	130
SOFT DRINK MIX			
Sugar-free			
all flavors	8 fl oz	0	4
Sugar-sweetened			
grape	8 fl oz	20	80
Rainbow punch	8 fl oz	21	80
Tropical punch	8 fl oz	21	80
Land O'Lakes			
chocolate milk			
homogenized	8 fl oz	26	210
low-fat (1%)	8 fl oz	26	160
skim	8 fl oz	26	140
eggnog	8 fl oz	32	300
fruit-flavored drinks	8 fl oz	27	120
Light 'n Juicy Juice Drinks			
grape, carton	6 fl oz	3	12
lemonade, carton	6 fl oz	1	5
orange, carton	6 fl oz	3	14
punch, carton	6 fl oz	3	12
Minute Maid			
FRUIT ADES			
grapeade, carton or from frozen concentrate	6 fl oz	13	94
lemonade or pink lemonade			
carton	6 fl oz	11	81
from frozen concentrate	6 fl oz	10	77
lemon/limeade, from frozen concentrate	6 fl oz	10	77
orangeade, from frozen concentrate	6 fl oz	11	85
FRUIT JUICES			
apple, carton or from frozen concentrate	6 fl oz	12	90
fruit punch, carton or from frozen concentrate	6 fl oz	12	91
grape, sweetened, from frozen concentrate	6 fl oz	13	98
grapefruit			
carton	6 fl oz	9	65
from frozen concentrate	6 fl oz	10	71

	Portion	Carbohydrates (g)	Total Calories
grapefruit, pink, from frozen concentrate	6 fl oz	10	71
lemon juice, from frozen concentrate	6 fl oz	3	22
orange			
regular, carton or from frozen concentrate	6 fl oz	11	82
calcium-fortified, carton or from frozen concentrate	6 fl oz	20	84
Country Style, carton or from frozen concentrate	6 fl oz	11	82
reduced-acid, from frozen concentrate	6 fl oz	11	82
pineapple, from frozen concentrate	6 fl oz	13	93
pineapple-orange, from frozen concentrate	6 fl oz	12	91
tangerine, sweetened, from frozen concentrate	6 fl oz	11	82

SOFT DRINKS

lemon-lime	6 fl oz	18	71
diet lemon-lime	6 fl oz	2	10
orange	6 fl oz	22	87
diet orange	6 fl oz	2	8

Mott's
JUICES

apple	6 oz	22	88
apple, natural	6 oz	19	76
apple cranberry	6 oz	24	83
apple grape	6 oz	23	86
apple raspberry	6 oz	22	83
grapefruit	10 oz	30	124
prune			
regular	6 oz	32	130
Country Style	6 oz	32	130

JUICE DRINKS

apple cranberry drink	10 oz	44	176
apple raspberry drink	10 oz	40	158
Beefamato	6 oz	19	80
Clamato	6 oz	23	96
fruit punch	10 oz	42	170
grape apple drink	10 oz	42	167
orange fruit juice blend	10 oz	35	144

Orange Plus
from frozen concentrate	6 fl oz	24	97

Ortega
Snap-E-Tom tomato cocktail	6 fl oz	7	40

	Portion	Carbohydrates (g)	Total Calories
Ovaltine Drink Mixes			
chocolate & malt	¾ oz dry mix	18	80
	¾ oz dry mix + 8 oz 2% milk	30	200
cocoa			
Hot 'n Rich	5 t	22	120
50-calorie	about 2½ t	8	50
sugar-free	about 2½ t	7	40
PDQ Drink Mixes			
chocolate	3–4 t + 8 oz whole milk	27	180
eggnog	2–3 t + 8 oz whole milk	39	230
strawberry	3–4 t + 8 oz whole milk	27	180
Pepsi			
Mountain Dew	6 fl oz	22	89
	12 fl oz	44	178
Pepsi-Cola	12 fl oz	39	156
Diet Pepsi	6 oz	tr	tr
Pepsi Light	6 oz	tr	1
Pepsi Free	6 oz	20	80
Diet Pepsi Free	6 oz	tr	tr
Slice	6 oz	20	76
Diet Slice	6 oz	3	13
Apple Slice	6 oz	24	98
Diet Apple Slice	6 oz	2	10
Cherry Cola Slice	6 oz	22	82
Diet Cherry Cola Slice	6 oz	2	10
Mandarin Orange Slice	6 oz	25	97
Diet Mandarin Orange Slice	6 oz	2	10
Perrier			
water, bottled	8 fl oz	0	0
Poland Spring			
water, bottled	1 c	0	0
Postum			
instant hot beverage, regular or coffee-flavored	6 fl oz	3	12
Royal Crown			
RC Cola	12 fl oz	39	156
RC 100	12 fl oz	39	156
Diet RC 100	12 fl oz	tr	1
Rose Holland *DRINK MIXES*			
Bloody Mary			
regular	1 fl oz	0	3
Smooth & Spicy	1 fl oz	0	1

	Portion	Carbohydrates (g)	Total Calories
Coco Casa			
cream of coconut	1 fl oz	17	78
piña colada	1 fl oz	16	88
strawberry colada	1 fl oz	17	78
daiquiri	1 fl oz	7	31
mai tai	1 fl oz	7	29
manhattan	1 fl oz	6	27
margarita	1 fl oz	6	25
old fashioned	1 fl oz	8	33
piña colada	1 fl oz	8	33
strawberry daiquiri	1 fl oz	6	27
strawberry margarita	1 fl oz	6	27
sweet & sour	1 fl oz	7	29
Tom Collins	1 fl oz	10	42
whiskey sour	1 fl oz	8	32

JUICE-FLAVORED DRINKS

	Portion	Carbohydrates (g)	Total Calories
grenadine	1 fl oz	16	64
lime juice	1 fl oz	10	41
Schweppes			
bitter lemon	6 oz	20	78
club soda	6 oz	tr	tr
Collins mixer	6 oz	17	70
ginger ale	6 oz	16	63
diet ginger ale	6 oz	tr	<2
ginger beer	6 oz	17	68
grapefruit	6 oz	19	77
grape soda	6 oz	23	92
lemon lime	6 oz	18	71
lemon sour	6 oz	19	75
root beer	6 oz	19	75
seltzer water (including flavored)	6 oz	19	75
sparkling orange	6 oz	22	86
tonic water	6 oz	16	64
diet tonic water	6 oz	tr	<2
Vichy water	6 oz	tr	tr
7-Up			
7-Up	6 oz	18	72
Diet 7-Up	6 oz	0	2
Cherry 7-Up	6 oz	19	74
Diet Cherry 7-Up	6 oz	tr	2
Sprite			
soda	12 fl oz	36	144
Sunrise			
flavored instant coffee	0.07 oz + 6 fl oz water	1	6

	Portion	Carbohydrates (g)	Total Calories
Tang			
breakfast beverage crystals, average of grape, grapefruit, & orange			
regular	6 fl oz	22	90
sugar-free	6 fl oz	1	6
V8			
vegetable juice			
regular	6 oz	8	35
no salt added	6 oz	9	40
Spicy Hot V8	6 oz	8	35

❏ BISCUITS *See* BREADS, ROLLS, BISCUITS, & MUFFINS

❏ BREADCRUMBS, CROUTONS, STUFFINGS, & SEASONED COATINGS

	Portion	Carbohydrates (g)	Total Calories
breadcrumbs			
enriched, dry, grated	1 c	73	390
white bread, enriched, soft	1 c	22	120
bread cubes, white, enriched	1 c	15	80
cornflake crumbs	1 oz	25	110
croutons, herb-seasoned	0.7 oz	14	70
stuffing, from mix			
bread	½ c	19	198
corn bread	½ c	23	117
enriched bread			
dry type	1 c	50	500
moist type	1 c	40	420

▪ BRAND NAME

	Portion	Carbohydrates (g)	Total Calories
Kellogg's			
cornflake crumbs	1 oz	25	110
Croutettes	0.7 oz dry	14	70
Nabisco			
cracker meal	2 T	12	50
Pepperidge Farm			
croutons	½ c	9	70
stuffings	1 oz	22	110
Pillsbury Stuffing Originals			
chicken	½ c	21	170
corn bread	½ c	25	170
mushroom	½ c	19	150

	Portion	Carbohydrates (g)	Cal
wild rice	½ c	21	160
Rice-A-Roni Stuffing Mixes			
bread/chicken flavor w/rice, prepared	½ c	20	240
bread/herb & butter & wild rice, prepared	½ c	20	240
bread w/wild rice, prepared	½ c	21	240
corn bread w/rice, prepared	½ c	21	240
Shake 'n Bake Seasoned Coatings			
Extra Crispy			
for chicken	¼ pouch	20	110
for pork	¼ pouch	21	120
Homestyle for chicken	¼ pouch	15	80
Stove Top			
FLEXIBLE SERVING STUFFING MIX			
chicken flavor, w/salted butter	½ c	20	170
corn bread flavor, w/salted butter	½ c	21	170
Homestyle herb, w/salted butter	½ c	20	170
STUFFING MIX			
Americana New England, w/ salted butter	½ c	21	180
Americana San Francisco, w/ salted butter	½ c	20	170
beef, w/salted butter	½ c	21	180
chicken flavor, w/salted butter	½ c	20	180
corn bread, w/salted butter	½ c	21	170
long grain & wild rice, w/salted butter	½ c	22	180
savory herbs, w/salted butter	½ c	20	180
turkey, w/salted butter	½ c	21	170
wild rice, w/salted butter	½ c	22	180

❑ BREADS, ROLLS, BISCUITS, & MUFFINS

Biscuits

	Portion	Carbohydrates (g)	Cal
baking powder, prepared w/ vegetable shortening			
from mix	1 (2″ diam)	14	95
from refrigerator dough	1 (2″ diam)	10	65
homemade	1 (2″ diam)	13	100
buttermilk, from refrigerator dough	2	18	130
flaky, from refrigerator dough	2	23	180

	Portion	Carbohydrates (g)	Total Calories
read & Bread Sticks			
Boston brown bread, canned	1.6 oz slice	21	95
bread sticks			
regular	1	5	23
garlic	1	4	24
sesame	1	4	56
Vienna	1	4	18
coffee cake *See* DESSERTS: CAKES, PASTRIES, & PIES			
corn bread			
from mix	2 oz	26	160
homemade			
w/enriched cornmeal	2.9 oz	29	198
w/whole-ground cornmeal	2.7 oz	24	172
cracked-wheat bread	1 lb loaf	227	1,190
	0.9 oz slice	12	65
danish *See* DESSERTS: CAKES, PASTRIES, & PIES			
French bread	1 lb loaf	230	1,270
	1.2 oz slice	18	100
fruit & nut quick bread, from mix	1.4 oz slice	22	118
honey wheatberry bread	1 oz slice	13	70
Italian bread	1 lb loaf	256	1,255
	1 oz slice	17	85
matzo *See* CRACKERS			
mixed-grain bread	1 lb loaf	212	1,165
	0.9 oz slice	12	65
oatmeal bread	1 lb loaf	212	1,145
	0.9 oz slice	12	65
pita bread, white	1 piece (6½″ diam)	33	165
pumpernickel bread	1 lb loaf	218	1,160
	1.1 oz slice	16	80
raisin bread	1 lb loaf	239	1,260
	0.9 oz slice	13	65
roman meal bread	1 oz slice	12	68
rye bread, light	1 lb loaf	218	1,190
	0.9 oz slice	12	65
sourdough bread	1 oz slice	13	68
Vienna bread	1 lb loaf	230	1,270
	0.9 oz slice	13	70
wheat bread	1 lb loaf	213	1,160
	0.9 oz slice	12	65
wheatberry bread	1 oz slice	12	70
white bread	1 lb loaf	222	1,210
	0.9 oz slice	12	65
	0.7 oz slice	10	55
whole-wheat bread	1 lb loaf	206	1,110
	1 oz slice	13	70

	Portion	Carbohydrates (g)	

Muffins

blueberry			
from mix	1.6 oz	22	14
homemade	1.6 oz	20	135
bran			
from mix	1.6 oz	24	140
homemade	1.6 oz	19	125
corn			
from mix	1.6 oz	22	145
homemade	1.6 oz	21	145
English			
regular	2 oz	27	140
sourdough	2 oz	25	129

Rolls & Bagels

bagel, plain or water, enriched	1 (3½" diam)	38	200
brown & serve roll	1	15	92
butterflake roll, from refrigerator dough	1	17	110
buttermilk roll, from mix	1	15	113
crescent roll, from refrigerator dough	2	24	200
croissant	2 oz	27	235
dinner roll			
commercial	1 oz	14	85
homemade	1.2 oz	20	120
frankfurter or hamburger roll	1.4 oz	20	115
French roll, enriched	1	28	137
hard roll, commercial	1.2 oz	30	155
hoagie or submarine roll	4.8 oz	72	400
parkerhouse roll	0.6 oz	8	59
popover			
from mix	1 oz	25	170
homemade	1.8 oz	13	112
raisin roll	2.1 oz	34	165
rye roll	0.6 oz	9	55
dark, hard	1 oz	15	80
light, hard	1 oz	14	79
sandwich roll	1.8 oz	28	162
sesame seed roll	0.6 oz	8	59
sweet roll See DESSERTS: CAKES, PASTRIES, & PIES			
wheat roll	0.6 oz	8	52
white roll			
from mix	2.2 oz	31	190
from refrigerator dough	1 oz	18	90
homemade	1.2 oz	20	119
whole-wheat roll, homemade	1.2 oz	18	90

	Portion	Carbohydrates (g)	Total Calories
...las			
tostada shell, corn	0.4 oz	7	50
...lla, corn	1.1 oz	13	65
...anned	1.2 oz	17	75
...ortilla, flour	1.1 oz	17	95

BRAND NAME

Lender's Bagels
all types	1	29–32	150–160

Ortega
taco/tostada shells	1	8	50

Pepperidge Farm
BREADS

cinnamon	2 slices	27	170
cracked-wheat	2 slices	26	140
Dijon rye	2 slices	27	160
Family pumpernickel	2 slices	30	160
honey bran	2 slices	36	190
honey wheatberry	2 slices	27	140
multigrain, very thin	2 slices	15	80
oatmeal	2 slices	25	140
Party Dijon Slices	4 slices	11	70
Party Pumpernickel Slices	4 slices	12	70
Party Rye Slices	4 slices	12	60
raisin w/cinnamon	2 slices	28	150
Sandwich White	2 slices	23	130
seeded Family rye	2 slices	16	80
seedless rye	2 slices	31	160
Toasting White	2 slices	32	170
wheat	2 slices	35	190
wheat germ	2 slices	25	130
white	2 slices	25	145
white, very thin	2 slices	16	80
whole-wheat	2 slices	24	130
whole-wheat, very thin	2 slices	15	80

ENGLISH MUFFINS

plain	1	26	140
cinnamon raisin	1	28	150

OLD FASHIONED MUFFINS, FROZEN

blueberry	1	27	170
bran w/raisins	1	27	170

	Portion	Carbohydrates (g)	Total Calories
carrot walnut	1	32	200
chocolate chip	1	31	210
cinnamon swirl	1	30	190
corn	1	27	180

ROLLS

butter crescent	1	13	110
club, brown & serve	1	20	100
French style	1	20	110
golden twist	1	13	110
hamburger	1	22	130
onion sandwich buns w/poppy seeds	1	26	150
parkerhouse	1	9	60
sourdough-style French	1	19	100

Pillsbury
BISCUITS

Big Country Southern Style	2	29	200
buttermilk	2	20	100
Country	2	20	100
Extra Lights flaky buttermilk	2	18	110
Hungry Jack			
buttermilk fluffy	2	24	180
extra rich buttermilk	2	19	110
flaky	2	24	170
Tenderflake baking powder dinner	2	14	110

BREAD STICKS

soft	1	17	100

DINNER ROLLS

butterflake	1	16	110
crescent	2	22	200

PIPIN' HOT DINNER ROLLS

Crusty French	1" slice	11	60
wheat	1" slice	12	80
white	1" slice	13	80

SWEET ROLLS & TURNOVERS See DESSERTS: CAKES, PASTRIES, & PIES

	Portion	Carbohydrates (g)	Total Calories

Sara Lee
BAGELS

plain	1	45	230
cinnamon & raisin	1	47	240
egg	1	46	240
onion	1	44	220
poppy seed	1	45	230

HEARTY FRUIT MUFFINS

apple cinnamon spice	1	36	220
banana nut bran	1	36	230
blueberry	1	34	200
oatmeal & fruit	1	36	230

L'ORIGINAL CROISSANTS

all butter	1	19	170
petite size	1	13	120
presliced	1	19	170
cheese	1	18	170
wheat & honey	1	18	170

LE PASTRIE CROISSANTS See DESSERTS: CAKES, PASTRIES, & PIES

LE SANDWICH CROISSANTS See ENTREES & MAIN COURSES, FROZEN

❑ BREAKFAST CEREALS, COLD & HOT

Cold Cereal

cornflakes, low-sodium	1 oz or about 1 c	25	113
crisp rice			
regular	1 oz or about 1 c	25	112
low-sodium	1 oz or about 1 c	26	114
granola, homemade	1 oz or about ¼ c	16	138
	1 c	67	595
oat flakes, fortified	1 oz or about ⅔ c	21	105
	1 c	35	177
rice, puffed	½ oz or about 1 c	13	57

	Portion	Carbohydrates (g)	Total Calories
wheat, puffed, plain	½ oz or about 1 c (heaping)	11	52
wheat, shredded			
large biscuit	1 rectangular	19	83
	2 round	30	133
small biscuit	1 oz or about ⅔ c	23	102
	⅞ oz box	20	89
wheat germ, toasted			
plain	1 oz or about ¼ c	14	108
	1 c	56	431
w/brown sugar & honey	1 oz or about ¼ c	17	107
	1 c	69	426

Hot Cereal

	Portion	Carbohydrates (g)	Total Calories
corn grits			
regular & quick			
dry	1 c	124	579
	1 T	8	36
cooked	1 c	31	146
	¾ c	24	110
instant, prepared			
plain	1 pkt	18	82
w/artificial cheese flavor	1 pkt	21	107
w/imitation bacon bits	1 pkt	22	104
w/imitation ham bits	1 pkt	21	103
farina			
dry	1 c	137	649
	1 T	9	40
cooked	1 c	25	116
	¾ c	19	87
grits; hominy grits See corn grits, *above*			
oats, regular, quick, & instant, nonfortified			
dry	⅓ c	18	104
cooked	1 c	25	145
	¾ c	19	108

▪ BRAND NAME

Arrowhead Mills
COLD CEREAL

	Portion	Carbohydrates (g)	Total Calories
Agrain & Agrain	2 oz	43	220
Arrowhead Crunch	1 oz	18	120
bran flakes	1 oz	20	100
corn, puffed	½ oz	11	50

	Portion	Carbohydrates (g)	Total Calories
cornflakes	1 oz	25	110
granola			
apple amaranth	2 oz	39	225
maple nut	2 oz	34	260
millet, puffed	½ oz	11	50
Nature O's	1 oz	20	110
rice, puffed	½ oz	12	50
wheat, puffed	½ oz	11	50
wheat bran	2 oz	30	200
wheat germ, raw	2 oz	26	210
HOT CEREAL			
Bear Mush	1 oz	21	100
corn grits			
white	2 oz	43	200
yellow	2 oz	44	200
4 Grain & Flax	2 oz	18	94
oat bran	1 oz	17	110
oatmeal, instant	1 oz	18	100
oats, steel cut	2 oz	37	220
Rice & Shine	¼ c	35	160
Seven Grain	1 oz	17	100
wheat, cracked	2 oz	40	180
Erewhon			
COLD CEREAL			
Crispy Brown Rice, regular or low-sodium	1 oz or about 1 c	24	110
Fruit 'n Wheat	1 oz or about ½ c	21	100
granola			
date nut	1 oz or about ¼ c	17	130
honey almond	1 oz or about ¼ c	17	130
maple	1 oz or about ¼ c	17	130
#9, w/bran, no salt added	1 oz or about ¼ c	17	130
spiced apple	1 oz or about ¼ c	17	130
Sunflower Crunch	1 oz or about ¼ c	18	130
raisin bran	1 oz or about ½ c	20	100
wheat flakes	1 oz or about ½ c	22	110

	Portion	Carbohydrates (g)	Total Calories
HOT CEREAL			
Barley Plus	1 oz or about ⅓ c dry	22	110
brown rice cream	1 oz or about ⅓ c dry	23	110
oat bran w/toasted wheat germ	1 oz or about ⅓ c dry	18	115
Featherweight Cold Cereal			
cornflakes	1¼ c	25	110
General Mills Cold Cereal			
Cheerios			
regular	1 oz or about 1¼ c	20	111
	¾ oz box	15	83
Honey Nut	1 oz or about ¾ c	23	107
	1 c	27	125
Crispy Wheats 'n Raisins	1 oz or about ¾ c	23	99
	1 c	35	150
Golden Grahams	1 oz or about ¾ c	24	109
	1 c	33	150
Kix	1 oz or about 1½ c	23	110
	¾ oz box	18	83
Lucky Charms	1 oz or about 1 c	23	110
Total	1 oz or about 1 c	22	100
Trix	1 oz or about 1 c	25	109
Wheaties	1 oz or about 1 c	23	99
Health Valley			
COLD CEREAL			
Amaranth Crunch w/raisins	1 oz or ¼ c	20	110
amaranth flakes	1 oz or ½ c	22	110
amaranth w/banana	1 oz or ¼ c	20	100
bran, w/apples & cinnamon or w/raisins	1 oz or ¼ c	21	100
Fiber 7 Flakes	1 oz or ½ c	22	100
Fruit Lites			
corn	½ oz or about ½ c	9	43
rice	½ oz or about ½ c	11	45
wheat	½ oz or about ½ c	11	43

	Portion	Carbohydrates (g)	Total Calories
granola *See* Real Granola, *below*			
Healthy Crunch, w/almonds & dates or w/apples & cinnamon	1 oz or about ¼ c	20	120
Lites			
corn or wheat, puffed	½ oz or about ½ c	11	50
rice, puffed	½ oz or about ½ c	12	50
oat bran flakes			
plain	1 oz or about ½ c	22	110
w/almonds & dates	1 oz or about ½ c	21	110
w/raisins	1 oz or about ½ c	22	107
Orangeola, w/almonds & dates or w/banana & Hawaiian fruit	1 oz or about ¼ c	19	120
raisin bran flakes	1 oz or about ½ c	24	110
Real Granola, w/almond crunch, w/Hawaiian fruit, or w/raisins & nuts	1 oz or about ¼ c	20	120
Sprouts 7, w/bananas & Hawaiian fruit or w/raisins	1 oz or about ¼ c	20	100
stoned-wheat flakes	1 oz or about ⅔ c	24	110
Swiss Breakfast, raisin nut or tropical fruit	1 oz or about ¼ c	19	100
wheat bran/Millers Flakes	2 oz	35	121
wheat germ w/fiber, almonds & dates or bananas & tropical fruit	1 oz or about ¼ c	20	100
HOT CEREAL			
hot oat bran w/apples	1 oz or about ¼ c	19	110
Heartland Cold Cereal			
Natural Cereal			
plain	1 oz or about ¼ c	19	123
	1 c	79	499
w/coconut	1 oz or about ¼ c	19	125
	1 c	71	463
w/raisins	1 oz or about ¼ c	20	120
	1 c	76	467

	Portion	Carbohydrates (g)	Total Calories
Kellogg's Cold Cereal			
All-Bran	1 oz or about ⅓ c	22	70
w/extra fiber	1 oz or about ½ c	22	60
w/fruit & almonds	1.3 oz or about ⅔ c	28	100
Apple Jacks	1 oz or about 1 c	26	110
Bran Buds	1 oz or about ⅓ c	22	70
bran flakes	1 oz or about ⅔ c	23	90
Cocoa Krispies	1 oz or about ¾ c	25	110
Corn Flakes			
regular	1 oz or about 1 c	25	110
honey & nut	1 oz or about ⅔ c	24	110
Corn Pops	1 oz or about 1 c	26	110
Cracklin' Oat Bran	1 oz or about ½ c	20	110
Crispix	1 oz or about 1 c	25	110
Froot Loops	1 oz or about 1 c	25	110
Frosted Flakes	1 oz or about ¾ c	26	110
Frosted Krispies	1 oz or about ¾ c	26	110
Frosted Mini-Wheats	1 oz = about 4 biscuits	24	100
Fruitful Bran	1.3 oz or about ⅔ c	30	120
Honey Smacks	1 oz or about ¾ c	25	110
Just Right			
all-grain	1 oz or about ⅔ c	24	100
w/fruit	1.3 oz or about ¾ c	30	140
Nutri-Grain			
almond raisin	1.4 oz or about ⅔ c	32	150
corn	1 oz or about ½ c	24	100

	Portion	Carbohydrates (g)	Total Calories
Nutri-Grain *(cont.)*			
wheat	1 oz or about ⅔ c	24	100
wheat & raisins	1.4 oz or about ⅔ c	32	130
Product 19	1 oz or about 1 c	24	110
raisin bran	1.4 oz or about ¾ c	30	120
Rice Krispies	1 oz or about 1 c	25	110
Special K	1 oz or about 1 c	20	110
Maltex Hot Cereal			
Maltex			
dry	¼ c	29	134
cooked	1 c	40	180
	¾ c	30	135
Old Fashioned Maltex	½ c cooked	15	77
Malt-O-Meal Hot Cereal			
Malt-O-Meal, plain or chocolate			
dry	1 T	8	38
cooked	1 c	26	122
	¾ c	19	92
Maypo			
Maypo			
dry	½ c	34	181
cooked	1 c	32	170
	¾ c	24	128
30-Second Oatmeal			
regular	½ c cooked	17	89
maple flavor	1 oz dry	19	101
Vermont-Style Hot Oat Cereal	½ c cooked	15	77
Nabisco			
COLD CEREAL			
Fruit Wheats, apple, raisin, or strawberry	1 oz	23	100
100% Bran	1 oz or about ½ c	21	76
	1 c	48	178
Shredded Wheat 'n Bran	1 oz	23	110
Team	1 oz or about 1 c	24	111
Toasted Wheat & Raisins	1 oz	23	100
HOT CEREAL			
Cream of Rice	1 oz dry	23	100
Cream of Wheat			
regular or instant	1 oz dry	22	100

	Portion	Carbohydrates (g)	Total Calories
Mix 'n Eat			
Original	1 oz dry	21	100
w/apple & cinnamon, w/ brown sugar cinnamon, or w/maple brown sugar	1¼ oz dry	30	130
w/peach or w/strawberry quick	1¼ oz dry	29	140
regular	1 oz dry	22	100
w/apples, raisins, & spice or w/maple brown sugar, artificially flavored	1 oz dry	24	110
Nature Valley Cold Cereal			
granola, toasted oat mixture	1 oz or about ⅓ c	19	126
	1 c	76	503
Post Cold Cereal			
Alpha-Bits	1 oz	24	110
Cocoa Pebbles	1 oz	25	110
C.W. Post Hearty Granola			
plain	1 oz	21	130
w/raisins	1 oz	21	120
Frosted Rice Krinkles	1 oz or about ⅞ c	26	109
Fruit & Fibre: dates, raisins, walnuts; Harvest Medley; Mountain Trail; or tropical fruit	1 oz	22	90
Fruity Pebbles	1 oz	25	110
granola See C.W. Post Hearty Granola, *above*			
Grape-Nuts			
regular	1 oz	23	110
raisin	1 oz	22	100
Grape-Nuts Flakes	1 oz	23	100
Honeycomb	1 oz	26	110
Natural Bran Flakes	1 oz	23	90
Natural Raisin Bran	1 oz	22	80
oat flakes, fortified	1 oz	20	110
Post Toasties	1 oz	24	110
Super Golden Crisp	1 oz or about ⅞ c	26	110
Quaker Oats			
COLD CEREAL			
bran, unprocessed	2 T	4	21
Cap'n Crunch			
regular	1 oz or about ¾ c	23	119
	1 c	30	156
w/Crunchberries	1 oz or about ¾ c	23	118
	1 c	29	146

	Portion	Carbohydrates (g)	Total Calories
Cap'n Crunch *(cont.)*			
peanut butter	1 oz or about ¾ c	22	124
	1 c	27	154
corn bran	1 oz or about ⅔ c	24	98
	1 c	30	124
King Vitaman	1 oz or about 1¼ c	24	115
	1 c	18	85
100% Natural Cereal			
plain	1 oz or about ¼ c	18	133
	1 c	65	489
w/apples & cinnamon	1 oz or about ¼ c	19	130
	1 c	70	478
w/raisins & dates	1 oz or about ¼ c	19	128
	1 c	72	496
Life, plain or cinnamon	1 oz or about ⅔ c	20	104
	1 c	32	162
Mr. T	1 c	23	121
Quisp	1 oz or about 1 c	24	117
HOT CEREAL			
farina, quick creamy wheat	2½ T un-cooked	22	101
oat bran	⅓ c uncooked	16	110
oatmeal, instant, prepared			
regular	1 pkt	18	105
w/apples & cinnamon	1 pkt	26	134
w/artificial maple & brown sugar	1 pkt	32	163
w/bran & raisins	1 pkt	29	153
w/cinnamon & spice	1 pkt	35	176
w/peaches & cream or w/ strawberries & cream, both artificially flavored	1 pkt	26	136
w/raisins & spice	1 pkt	31	159
w/raisins, dates, & walnuts	1 pkt	25	150
w/real honey & graham	1 pkt	27	136
Quaker Oats, Quick & Old Fashioned	⅓ c dry or ⅔ c cooked	18	109
Whole Wheat Hot Natural	⅓ c dry or ⅔ c cooked	22	106

	Portion	Carbohydrates (g)	Total Calories
Ralston Purina			
COLD CEREAL			
Bran Chex	1 oz or about ⅔ c	23	91
	1 c	39	156
Cookie-Crisp	1 oz or about 1 c	25	114
Corn Chex	1 oz or about 1 c	25	111
	¾ oz box	19	84
cornflakes	1 oz or about 1 c	25	111
40% bran flakes	1 oz or about ¾ c	23	92
	1 c	39	159
raisin bran	1⅓ oz or about ¾ c	31	120
	1 c	47	178
Rice Chex	1 oz or about 1⅛ c	25	112
	⅞ oz box	22	98
sugar frosted flakes	1 oz or about ¾ c	26	111
	1 c	34	149
Tasteeos	1 oz or about 1¼ c	22	111
	1 c	19	94
Waffelos	1 oz or about 1 c	25	115
Wheat Chex	1 oz or about ⅔ c	23	104
	1 c	38	169
Wheat 'n Raisin Chex	1⅓ oz or about ¾ c	30	130
	1 c	43	185
HOT CEREAL			
Ralston			
dry	¼ c	22	102
cooked	1 c	28	134
	¾ c	21	100
Roman Meal Hot Cereal			
Roman Meal			
plain			
dry	⅓ c	22	100
cooked	1 c	33	147
	¾ c	25	111
w/oats			
dry	¼ c	17	85
cooked	1 c	34	169
	¾ c	26	127

	Portion	Carbohydrates (g)	Total Calories
Sun Country Granola			
w/almonds	1 oz	19	130
w/raisins or w/raisins & dates	1 oz	20	130
Sunshine			
shredded wheat			
regular	1 biscuit	19	90
bite size	⅔ c	22	110
U.S. Mills			
See also Erewhon, *above*			
Skinner's raisin bran	1 oz or about ½ c	20	100
Uncle Sam, laxative	1 oz or about ½ c	19	110
Wheatena			
Wheatena			
dry	¼ c	27	125
cooked	1 c	29	135
	¾ c	22	101

❏ BREAKFAST FOODS, PREPARED

See also EGGS & EGG SUBSTITUTES; FAST FOODS

French toast, homemade	1 slice	17	155
pancakes			
from mix			
plain	1 (4″ diam)	8	60
buckwheat	1 (4″ diam)	6	55
extra light	3 (4″ diam)	28	200
homemade			
plain	1 (4″ diam)	9	60
cornmeal	1 (4″ diam)	11	68
soy	1 (4″ diam)	10	68
waffles			
from mix	1 (7″ diam)	27	205
frozen	1	14	95
homemade	1 (7″ diam)	26	245

▪ BRAND NAME

Arrowhead Mills Pancake Mixes			
Blue Heaven	½ c	40	200
buckwheat	½ c	53	270
Griddle Lite	½ c	50	260
multigrain	½ c	70	350
triticale	½ c	53	270

	Portion	Carbohydrates (g)	Total Calories
Aunt Jemima			
FRENCH TOAST, FROZEN			
plain	2 slices	27	168
cinnamon swirl	2 slices	28	190
raisin	2 slices	29	185
PANCAKE & WAFFLE MIXES			
original flavor	¼ c	23	108
buckwheat	¼ c	21	107
buttermilk	⅓ c	37	175
whole-wheat	⅓ c	29	142
PANCAKE BATTER, FROZEN			
original flavor	3 (4″ diam)	42	210
blueberry	3 (4″ diam)	42	205
buttermilk	3 (4″ diam)	43	212
PANCAKES, FROZEN			
original flavor	3 (4″ diam)	47	246
blueberry	3 (4″ diam)	46	249
buttermilk	3 (4″ diam)	45	240
WAFFLES, FROZEN			
original flavor	2	29	173
apple & cinnamon	2	29	173
blueberry	2	29	173
buttermilk	2	29	175
Fearn Pancake Mixes			
buckwheat	½ c dry	44	235
Rich Earth	½ c dry	41	190
7-grain buttermilk	½ c dry	38	200
stone-ground whole-wheat	½ c dry	43	220
unbleached wheat & soya	½ c dry	46	235
Featherweight			
pancake mix	3 (4″ diam)	24	130
Health Valley			
7 Sprouted Grains buttermilk pancake & biscuit mix	1 oz	22	100
Kellogg's			
EGGO FROZEN WAFFLES			
apple cinnamon	1	18	130
buttermilk	1	16	120
Homestyle	1	16	120

POP-TARTS See DESSERTS: CAKES, PASTRIES, & PIES

Nabisco Toastettes *See* DESSERTS: CAKES, PASTRIES, & PIES

	Portion	Carbohydrates (g)	Total Calories
Swanson			
GREAT STARTS BREAKFASTS			
French toast (cinnamon swirl)	6½ oz	40	480
French toast w/sausages	6½ oz	38	460
omelets w/cheese sauce & ham	7 oz	14	400
pancakes & blueberry sauce	7 oz	71	410
pancakes & sausages	6 oz	53	470
scrambled eggs & sausage w/ hashed brown potatoes	6¼ oz	17	430
Spanish-style omelet	7¾ oz	15	250
GREAT STARTS BREAKFAST SANDWICHES			
biscuit & sausage	4¾ oz	35	410
egg, Canadian bacon, & cheese/muffin	4½ oz	27	310
sausage, egg, & cheese/biscuit	6¼ oz	37	520
steak, egg, & cheese/muffin	5¼ oz	27	390

❏ BROWNIES *See* COOKIES, BARS, & BROWNIES

❏ BUTTER & MARGARINE SPREADS

Butter

See also NUTS & NUT-BASED BUTTERS, FLOURS, MEALS, MILKS, PASTES, & POWDERS; SEEDS & SEED-BASED BUTTERS, FLOURS, & MEALS

	Portion	Carbohydrates (g)	Total Calories
salted or unsalted	1 t	tr	36
	1 stick = 4 oz or about ½ c	tr	813
whipped, salted	1 t	tr	27
	1 stick = 4 oz or about ½ c	tr	542

Margarine

REGULAR

Hard, Stick or Brick

	Portion	Carbohydrates (g)	Total Calories
all kinds	1 stick	1	815
	1 t	0	34

	Portion	Carbohydrates (g)	Total Calories
Liquid, Bottle			
soybean (hydrogenated), soybean, & cottonseed	1 c 1 t	0 0	1,637 34
Soft, Tub			
all kinds	1 c 1 t	1–2 0	1,626 34
IMITATION (ABOUT 40% FAT)			
all kinds	1 c 1 t	1 0	801 17
SPREAD, MARGARINELIKE (ABOUT 60% FAT)			
all kinds, stick or tub	1 c 1 t	0 0	1,236 26

• BRAND NAME

Blue Bonnet Margarine

Butter Blend, soft or stick, salted or unsalted	1 T	0	90
margarine			
regular, soft or stick	1 T	0	100
diet	1 T	0	50
whipped, soft or stick	1 T	0	70
spread			
Light Tasty, 52% vegetable oil	1 T	0	60
52% fat	1 T	0	80
stick, 70% or 75% fat	1 T	0	90
whipped, 60% fat	1 T	0	50

Fleischmann's

margarine			
regular: stick, soft, or squeeze; salted or unsalted	1 T	0	100
diet or diet w/lite salt	1 T	0	50
whipped, salted or unsalted	1 T	0	70
spread, light corn oil, soft or stick	1 T	0	80

Land O'Lakes

butter			
regular, salted or unsalted	1 T	0	100
whipped, salted or unsalted	1 T	0	60
Country Morning Blend margarine			
stick, salted or unsalted	1 T	0	100
soft, tub, salted or unsalted	1 T	0	90

	Portion	Carbohydrates (g)	Total Calories
margarine, stick or soft tub, regular (soy oil) or premium (corn oil)	1 T	0	100
Mazola			
margarine, regular, salted or unsalted	1 T	0	100
diet margarine	1 T	0	50
Nucoa			
margarine	1 T	0	100
soft margarine	1 T	0	90

❏ CAKES *See* DESSERTS: CAKES, PASTRIES, & PIES

❏ CANDIED FRUIT *See* BAKING INGREDIENTS

❏ CANDY

butterscotch	6 pieces	24	116
butterscotch chips	1 oz	19	150
caramels			
plain or chocolate	3	22	112
plain or chocolate w/nuts	2	20	120
chocolate			
chocolate fudge center	1	22	129
chocolate fudge w/nuts center	1	19	127
coconut center	1	20	123
cream center	1	19	102
fondant center	1	23	115
vanilla cream center	1	18	114
chocolate chips			
chocolate-flavored	¼ c	32	195
dark	1 oz	18	148
milk chocolate	¼ c	27	218
semisweet	1 c or 6 oz (60 chips/oz)	97	860
chocolate-covered almonds	1 oz	11	159
chocolate-covered Brazil nuts	1 oz	9	162
chocolate-covered peanuts	1 oz	13	153
chocolate-covered raisins	1 oz	20	115
chocolate kisses	6	16	154
chocolate stars	7	17	145
English toffee	1 oz	10	193

	Portion	Carbohydrates (g)	Total Calories
fondant, uncoated (mints, candy corn, other)	1 oz	27	105
fudge			
chocolate, plain	1 oz	21	115
chocolate w/nuts	1 oz	19	119
vanilla	1 oz	21	111
vanilla w/nuts	1 oz	19	119
granola bars See COOKIES, BARS, & BROWNIES			
gum drops	1 oz	25	100
hard candy	1 oz	28	110
	6 pieces	27	108
jelly beans	1 oz	26	105
	10	17	66
lollipop	1 medium	28	108
malted milk balls	14	18	135
marshmallows	1 oz	23	90
	1 large	6	25
mints	14	26	104
peanut brittle	1 oz	20	123
sugar-coated almonds	7	20	128

• BRAND NAME

NOTE: Candies may be listed under product name (e.g., Milky Way) or company name (e.g., Cadbury or Hershey).

	Portion	Carbohydrates (g)	Total Calories
Almond Joy	1 oz	19	151
Baby Ruth	½ bar	18	130
Baker's chocolate See BAKING INGREDIENTS			
Beechies candy-coated gum, all flavors	1 piece	2	6
Beech-Nut			
cough drops, all flavors	1	3	10
gum, all flavors	1 piece	2	10
Bit-O-Honey	1 oz	21	121
	1.8 oz	39	220
Bonkers!, all flavors	1 piece	5	20
Breath Savers Mints, sugar-free, all flavors	1	2	8
Bubble Yum bubble gum, all flavors			
regular	1 piece	7	25
sugarless	1 piece	5	20
Butterfinger	½ bar	19	130
Butter Nut	1.8 oz	29	250
Cadbury			
chocolate almond	1 oz	16	155
chocolate Brazil nut	1 oz	15	156

	Portion	Carbohydrates (g)	Total Calories
Cadbury *(cont.)*			
chocolate hazelnut	1 oz	16	155
chocolate Krisp	1 oz	18	146
creme eggs	1 oz	19	136
fruit & nut	1 oz	16	152
milk chocolate	1 oz	17	151
Caramello	1 oz	17	144
Caravelle	1 oz	21	137
Care-Free			
sugarless bubble gum, all flavors	1 piece	2	10
sugarless gum, all flavors	1 piece	2	8
Charleston Chew!	½ piece	22	120
Chunky			
Original	1 oz	18	143
milk chocolate	1 oz	18	120
peanut	1 oz	16	151
pecan	1 oz	18	148
Fruit Stripe			
bubble gum, all flavors	1 piece	2	10
gum, all flavors	1 piece	2	10
Good 'n Fruity	1½ oz	40	160
Good & Plenty	1½ oz	37	151
Hershey			
chocolate chips & unsweetened chocolate *See* BAKING INGREDIENTS			
chocolate Kisses	9 or 1.46 oz	23	220
Krackel	1.6 oz	28	250
milk chocolate	1.65 oz	27	250
milk chocolate w/almonds	1.55 oz	22	250
Special Dark sweet chocolate	1.45 oz	25	220
Junior Mints	12	24	120
Kit Kat	1.6 oz	29	250
Life Savers			
lollipops, all flavors	1	11	45
milk chocolate stars	13	19	160
roll candy, all flavors, regular or sugar-free	1 piece	2	8
M&M's			
regular	1.59 oz	28	220
peanut	1.67 oz	28	240
Marathon	1.38 oz	27	179
Mars	1.7 oz	29	230
Milk Mounds	1 oz	16	138
Milk Shake	2 oz	43	250
Milky Way	2.1 oz	43	260
Mounds	1 oz	20	147
Mr. Goodbar	1.85 oz	24	300
Nestlé			
Crunch	1.06 oz	19	160
milk chocolate	1.07 oz	19	160
milk chocolate w/almonds	1 oz	16	150

	Portion	Carbohydrates (g)	Total Calories
Oh Henry!	1 oz	16	139
Pay Day	1.9 oz	28	250
Pearson's			
Carmel Nip	4	23	120
Coffee Nip	4	23	120
Licorice Nip	4	23	120
Chocolate Parfait	4	23	120
Peppermint Pattie	1 oz	25	124
Pillsbury food sticks	4	27	180
Planters			
peanut bar			
regular or honey roasted	1.6 oz	25	230
Sweet 'n Crunchy	1.6 oz	21	250
Old Fashioned peanut candy	1 oz	13	140
Pom Poms	½ box	15	100
Power House	1 oz	19	131
Reese's			
Peanut Butter Cup	1.8 oz	26	280
peanut butter–flavored chips	¼ c	19	223
Pieces	1.95 oz	34	270
Rolo	9 pieces or 1.93 oz	37	270
Skor	1.4 oz	22	220
Snickers	2 oz	33	270
Sno-Caps	1 oz	22	132
Starbar	1 oz	16	141
Sugar Babies	1 pkg	40	180
Sugar Daddy	1	33	150
Summit	0.76 oz	11	100
Thousand Dollar	1½ oz	31	200
Three Musketeers	2.28 oz	49	280
Twix	1.73 oz	16	120
Whatchamacallit	1.8 oz	29	270
Y&S Bites or Twizzlers	1 oz	23	100
Zero	2 oz	42	250

❏ **CANNED MEATS** *See* PROCESSED MEAT & POULTRY PRODUCTS

❏ **CEREAL, BREAKFAST** *See* BREAKFAST CEREALS, COLD & HOT

	Portion	Carbohydrates (g)	Total Calories

❑ CHEESE & CHEESE FOODS

Natural Cheese

	Portion	Carbohydrates (g)	Total Calories
bleu	1 oz	tr	100
	1 c, crumbled, not packed	3	477
brick	1″ cube	tr	64
	1 oz	tr	105
Brie	1 oz	tr	95
	4½ oz	tr	427
Camembert	1 oz	tr	85
	3⅓ oz	tr	114
caraway	1 oz	1	107
cheddar	1 oz	tr	114
	1 c, shredded, not packed	1	455
Cheshire	1 oz	1	110
Colby	1″ cube	tr	68
	1 oz	tr	112
cottage			
creamed, small curd	4 oz	3	117
	1 c, not packed	6	217
fruit added	4 oz	15	140
	1 c, not packed	30	279
dry curd	4 oz	2	96
	1 c, not packed	3	123
low-fat			
2%	4 oz	4	101
	1 c, not packed	8	203
1%	4 oz	3	82
	1 c, not packed	6	164
cream	1 oz	tr	99
	3 oz	2	297
Edam	1 oz	tr	101
	7 oz	3	706
feta, from sheep's milk	1 oz	1	75
fontina	1 oz	tr	110
	8 oz	4	883
gjetost, from goats' & cows' milk	1 oz	12	132
	8 oz	97	1,057
Gouda	1 oz	tr	101
	7 oz	4	705
Gruyère	1 oz	tr	117
	6 oz	tr	702

	Portion	Carbohydrates (g)	Total Calories
Limburger	1 oz	tr	93
	8 oz	1	742
Monterey Jack	1 oz	tr	106
	6 oz	1	635
mozzarella	1 oz	tr	80
low-moisture	1″ cube	tr	56
	1 oz	1	90
part skim	1″ cube	tr	49
	1 oz	1	79
part skim	1 oz	1	72
Muenster	1 oz	tr	104
	6 oz	2	626
Neufchâtel	1 oz	1	74
	3 oz	2	221
Parmesan			
grated	1 T	tr	23
	1 oz	1	129
hard	1 oz	1	111
	5 oz	5	557
Port du Salut	1 oz	tr	100
	6 oz	1	598
provolone	1 oz	1	100
	6 oz	4	598
ricotta			
whole milk	½ c	4	216
part skim milk	½ c	6	171
Romano, hard	1 oz	1	110
	5 oz	5	549
Roquefort, from sheep's milk	1 oz	tr	105
	3 oz	2	314
Swiss	1″ cube	1	56
	1 oz	1	107
Tilsit	1 oz	1	96
	6 oz	3	578

whey *See* MILK, MILK SUBSTITUTES, & MILK PRODUCTS

Process Cheese & Cheese Food

CHEESE FOOD

American			
cold pack	1 oz	2	94
	8 oz	19	752
pasteurized process	1 oz	2	93
	8 oz	17	745
Swiss, pasteurized process	1 oz	1	92
	8 oz	10	734

CHEESE SPREAD

American, pasteurized process	1 oz	2	82
	5 oz	12	412

	Portion	Carbohydrates (g)	Total Calories
PASTEURIZED PROCESS CHEESE			
American	1″ cube	tr	66
	1 oz	tr	106
pimiento	1″ cube	tr	66
	1 oz	tr	106
Swiss	1″ cube	tr	60
	1 oz	1	95

▪ BRAND NAME

Armour
cheddar, regular or lower salt	1 oz	1	110
Colby, regular or lower salt	1 oz	1	110
Monterey Jack, regular or lower salt	1 oz	1	110

Bonbel *See* Fromageries Bel, *below*
Delicia Pasteurized Process Cheese Substitute
American	1 oz	1	80
American w/peppers	1 oz	1	80
Hickory Smoked American	1 oz	0	80

Featherweight
cheddar, low-sodium	1 oz	1	110

Friendship
cottage cheese			
California style, 4% milk fat	½ c	4	120
Friendship 'n Fruit	6 oz	23	100
low-fat			
regular or lactose-reduced, both 1% milk fat	½ c	4	90
large curd pot style, 2% milk fat	½ c	4	100
w/pineapple, 4% milk fat	½ c	15	140
cream cheese	1 oz	1	103
farmer cheese	½ c	4	160
natural hoop cheese, ½% milk fat	4 oz	2	84

Fromageries Bel
Babybel	1 oz	tr	91
Bombino	1 oz	tr	103
Bonbel	1 oz	tr	100
cheddar	1 oz	tr	110
Edam	1 oz	tr	100
Gouda	1 oz	tr	110
Mini Babybel	¾ oz	tr	74
Mini Bonbel	¾ oz	tr	74
Mini Gouda	¾ oz	tr	80
Reduced Mini	¾ oz	tr	45

	Portion	Carbohydrates (g)	Total Calories
Hoffman's			
CHEESE FOOD			
American	1 oz	3	100
Chees'n Bacon	1 oz	3	90
Chees'n Onion	1 oz	3	100
Chees'n Salami	1 oz	3	90
Hot Pepper w/jalapeño peppers	1 oz	2	90
Swisson Rye w/caraway	1 oz	2	90
PASTEURIZED PROCESS CHEESE			
American	1 oz	1	110
cheddar			
Smokey Sharp	1 oz	1	110
Super Sharp	1 oz	2	110
Smokey Swiss'n Cheddar	1 oz	1	110
Land O'Lakes			
CULTURED CHEESE			
cottage cheese	4 oz	3	120
cottage cheese, 2% milk fat	4 oz	4	100
NATURAL CHEESE			
brick	1 oz	1	110
cheddar	1 oz	<1	110
Colby	1 oz	1	110
Edam	1 oz	<1	100
Gouda	1 oz	1	100
Monterey Jack	1 oz	<1	110
mozzarella, low-moisture, part skim	1 oz	1	80
Muenster	1 oz	<1	100
provolone	1 oz	1	100
Swiss	1 oz	1	110
PROCESS CHEESE & CHEESE FOOD			
American	1 oz	<1	110
Golden Velvet cheese spread	1 oz	2	80
jalapeño cheese food	1 oz	2	90
onion cheese food	1 oz	2	90
pepperoni cheese food	1 oz	1	90
Laughing Cow			
average values of cheese spreads	1 oz	1	78
May-Bud			
Edam	1 oz	0	100
farmers, semisoft, part skim	1 oz	1	90
Gouda	1 oz	1	100
Monterey Jack	1 oz	0	110

	Portion	Carbohydrates (g)	Total Calories
Nabisco Easy Cheese			
pasteurized process cheese spread, all flavors	1 oz	2	80
Wispride Cold Pack Cheese Food			
port wine	1 oz	3	100
sharp cheddar	1 oz	2	100

❑ **CHICKEN** *See* POULTRY, FRESH & PROCESSED

❑ **CHUTNEYS** *See* PICKLES, OLIVES, RELISHES, & CHUTNEYS

❑ **COATINGS, SEASONED** *See* BREADCRUMBS, CROUTONS, STUFFINGS, & SEASONED COATINGS

❑ **CONDIMENTS** *See* SAUCES, GRAVIES, & CONDIMENTS

❑ **COOKIES, BARS, & BROWNIES**

animal cookies	15	22	120
arrowroot cookies	2	7	47
brownies			
butterscotch	1 oz	16	115
chocolate, from mix	1.1 oz	20	130
chocolate, w/nuts			
commercial, frosted	0.9 oz	16	100
homemade, w/vegetable oil	0.7 oz	11	95
cherry coolers	2	9	58
chocolate chip cookies			
commercial	4 (2¼″ diam)	28	180
from refrigerator dough	4 (2¼″ diam)	32	225
homemade, w/vegetable shortening	4 (2⅓″ diam)	26	185
w/coconut	1	10	82
chocolate cookies	1	15	93
chocolate sandwich cookies	1	7	49
chocolate snaps	4	9	53
coconut bars	1	14	109
fig bars	4 = 2 oz	42	210

	Portion	Carbohydrates (g)	Total Calories
gingersnaps			
commercial	3 small	10	50
homemade	1	5	34
golden fruit cookies	1	15	63
graham crackers	2	11	60
chocolate-covered	1	9	62
granola bars	1	16	109
lemon coolers	2	9	57
macaroons	1	9	67
molasses cookies	1	10	71
oatmeal cookies			
from mix	2	17	130
homemade	1	9	62
oatmeal chocolate chip cookies	1	7	57
oatmeal raisin cookies			
from refrigerator dough	1	9	61
homemade	4 (2⅝" diam)	36	245
peanut butter bars	1	26	198
peanut butter cookies			
from refrigerator dough	1	6	50
homemade	4 = 1.7 oz	28	245
peanut cookies	1	8	57
sandwich-type cookies, chocolate or vanilla	4 = 1.4 oz	29	195
shortbread cookies			
commercial	4 small	20	155
homemade, w/margarine	2 large	17	145
social tea cookies	2	8	43
sugar cookies			
from mix	2	18	120
from refrigerator dough	4 = 1.7 oz	31	235
homemade	1	14	89
sugar wafers	2	8	53
vanilla cream sandwich cookies	1	10	69
vanilla wafers	10 = 1.4 oz	29	185
Vienna dream bars, from mix	1	10	90
Vienna finger sandwich cookies	1	11	72

• BRAND NAME

Famous Amos

chocolate chip, no nuts, extra chips	1 oz	17	147
chocolate chip w/macadamia nuts	1 oz	16	152
chocolate chip w/pecans	1 oz	17	151
oatmeal w/cinnamon & raisins	1 oz	19	133

	Portion	Carbohydrates (g)	Total Calories
Health Valley			
Animal Snaps, cinnamon or vanilla	6	3	15
fruit bars, apple, date, or raisin	2	33	180
Fruit Jumbos			
almonds & dates or raisins & nuts	1	12	85
oat bran	1	12	80
tropical fruit	1	12	85
graham crackers			
amaranth	3	11	50
oat bran	3	9	54
Jumbos			
amaranth	1	14	60
cinnamon	1	10	70
oatmeal	1	10	60
peanut butter	1	11	70
tofu cookies	4	6	52
wheat-free cookies	4	7	52
Hershey New Trail Granola Snack Bars			
chocolate chip	1	23	190
chocolate-covered cocoa creme	1	21	200
chocolate-covered honey graham	1	21	200
chocolate-covered peanut butter	1	20	200
peanut butter	1	21	190
peanut butter & chocolate chip	1	21	180
Kellogg's Rice Krispies Bars			
chocolate chip	1	21	120
Cocoa Krispies chocolate chip	1	22	120
raisin	1	22	120
Nabisco			
Almost Home Family-Style cookies			
fudge chocolate chip cookies	2	20	130
fudge & nut brownies	1	23	160
fudge & vanilla creme sandwiches	1	20	140
iced Dutch apple fruit sticks	1	14	70
oatmeal raisin cookies	2	20	130
peanut butter chocolate chip cookies	2	16	140
Real chocolate chip cookies	2	20	130
Old Fashioned sugar cookies	2	20	130
Apple Newtons	1	21	110
Barnum's Animals (animal crackers)	11	21	130
Bugs Bunny graham cookies	9	20	120
Cameo creme sandwiches	2	21	140

	Portion	Carbohydrates (g)	Tota Calori
Chewy Chips Ahoy!	2	18	130
Chips 'n More	2	18	150
chocolate grahams	3	19	150
chocolate snaps	7	21	130
Cinnamon Treats	2	11	60
Cookies 'n Fudge	3	18	150
devil's food cakes	1	23	110
Famous chocolate wafers	5	21	130
Giggles vanilla sandwich cookies	2	17	140
graham or Honey Maid graham crackers	2	11	60
imported Danish cookies	5	18	150
I Screams n' You Screams Double Dip chocolate creme sandwiches	2	20	150
Lorna Doone shortbread	4	18	140
Mallomars	2	18	130
National arrowroot biscuits	6	21	130
Old Fashion ginger snaps	4	22	120
Oreo chocolate sandwich cookies	3	20	140
Oreo mint creme chocolate sandwich cookies	2	20	150
Pantry molasses cookies	2	21	130
pecan shortbread cookies	2	16	150
Pinwheels	1	20	130
Social Tea biscuits	6	21	130
Pepperidge Farm _ASSORTMENT COOKIES_			
Champagne	2	14	110
Original Pirouettes	2	11	110
Seville	2	12	100
DISTINCTIVE COOKIES			
Bordeaux	3	16	110
Brussels	3	21	170
Chessmen	3	19	130
Geneva	3	21	190
Lido	2	21	180
Milano	3	15	130
Nassau	2	19	170
Orleans	3	11	100
FRUIT COOKIES			
apricot-raspberry	3	24	150
KITCHEN HEARTH COOKIES			
date nut granola	3	21	170
raisin bran	3	22	160

	Portion	Carbohydrates (g)	Total Calories
OLD FASHIONED COOKIES			
brownie chocolate nut	3	19	170
chocolate chip	3	20	150
chocolate chocolate chip	3	19	160
Gingerman	3	16	100
hazelnut	3	21	170
Irish oatmeal	3	21	150
Lemon Nut Crunch	3	20	180
Molasses Crisps	3	13	100
oatmeal raisin	3	23	170
shortbread	3	15	130
sugar	3	21	150
SPECIAL COLLECTION COOKIES			
Almond Supreme	2	13	140
Chocolate Chunk Pecan	2	15	130
milk chocolate macadamia	2	15	140
Pillsbury			
chocolate chip cookies	3	29	210
fudge brownies	1	22	140
oatmeal raisin cookies	3	28	200
peanut butter cookies	3	28	200
sugar cookies	3	30	200
Quaker Oats			
CHEWY GRANOLA BARS			
chocolate chip	1	19	129
chocolate, graham, & marshmallow	1	20	126
chunky nut & raisin	1	17	133
honey & oats	1	19	125
peanut butter	1	18	130
raisin & cinnamon	1	19	130
GRANOLA DIPPS BARS			
chocolate chip	1	18	138
honey & oats	1	19	137
peanut butter	1	17	141
raisin & almond	1	19	139
Rokeach			
graham crackers	8	21	120
Sunshine			
animal crackers	14	22	120
butter-flavored cookies	4	17	120
Chip-A-Roos	2	16	130
Chips 'n Middles	2	19	140
chocolate fudge sandwiches	2	18	150
cinnamon graham crackers	4, after breaking	11	70

	Portion	Carbohydrates (g)	Calc
Country Style oatmeal cookies	2	16	110
fig bars	2	22	90
ginger snaps	5	16	100
Golden Fruit raisin biscuits	2, after breaking	29	150
honey graham crackers	4, after breaking	10	60
Hydrox	3	21	160
Mallopuffs	2	24	140
sugar wafers	3	18	130
vanilla wafers	6	18	130
Vienna fingers	2	21	140

❑ CORNMEAL *See* FLOURS & CORNMEALS

❑ CRACKERS
See also SNACKS

bread sticks *See* BREADS, ROLLS, BISCUITS, & MUFFINS			
cheese, plain	10 (1″ square)	6	50
cheese & peanut butter sandwich	1	5	40
graham *See* COOKIES, BARS, & BROWNIES			
matzo	1	25	117
melba toast, plain	1	4	20
oyster	33	20	120
rusk	1	7	42
rye crisp	2 triple crackers	10	50
rye wafers, whole-grain	2 = ½ oz	10	55
saltines	4	9	50
snack-type crackers, standard, round	1	2	15
soda, unsalted tops	10	20	120
taco shells *See* BREADS, ROLLS, BISCUITS, & MUFFINS			
tortillas *See* BREADS, ROLLS, BISCUITS, & MUFFINS			
wheat, thin	4	5	35
whole-wheat wafers	2	5	35
zwieback *See* INFANT & TODDLER FOODS			

▪ BRAND NAME

Cracottes

regular or salt-free	1	3	12
whole-wheat	1	3	13

	Portion	Carbohydrates (g)	Total Calories
Featherweight			
crackers	2	5	30
wafers			
bran	4	8	50
wheat	4	9	50
Health Valley			
Cheese Wheels	12	14	140
French onion, regular or no salt	13	16	130
herb, regular or no salt	13	16	130
honey graham	13	16	130
sesame, regular or no salt	13	16	130
7-Grain Vegetable			
regular	1 oz	16	130
no salt	1 oz	17	120
stoned-wheat, regular or no salt	13	16	130
Nabisco			
Bacon-Flavored Thins	7	8	70
Better Blue Cheese	10	8	70
Better Cheddars	11	8	70
Better Cheddars 'n' Bacon	10	8	70
Better Nacho	9	8	70
Better Swiss Cheese	10	8	70
cheese peanut butter sandwich	2	8	70
Cheese Tid-Bits	16	8	70
Cheese Wheat Thins	9	9	70
Chicken in a Biskit	7	8	70
Crown Pilot	1	11	60
Dandy Soup & Oyster	20	10	60
Dip in a Chip Cheese 'n Chive	8	8	70
Escort	3	9	80
graham or Honey Maid graham crackers *See* COOKIES, BARS, & BROWNIES			
Great Crisps! *See* SNACKS			
Holland Rusk	1	10	60
Meal Mates	3	9	70
Nips *See* SNACKS			
Nutty Wheat Thins	7	8	80
Oysterettes	18	10	60
Premium saltines, regular or low-salt	5	10	60
Ritz			
regular or low-salt	4	9	70
cheese	5	8	70
Royal Lunch Milk	1	10	60
Sea Rounds	1	10	60
Sociables	6	9	70
Toasted Peanut Butter Sandwich	2	8	70

	Portion	Carbohydrates (g)	Total Calories
Triscuits, regular or low-salt	3	10	60
Twigs, sesame or cheese	5	8	70
Uneeda Biscuit, unsalted tops	3	10	60
Vegetable Thins	7	8	70
Waverly	4	10	70
Wheatsworth	5	9	70
Wheat Thins, regular or low-salt	8	9	70
Pepperidge Farm			
butter-flavored thin crackers	4	10	80
English water biscuits	4	13	70
Hearty wheat crackers	4	13	100
sesame crackers	4	11	80
Snack Sticks See SNACKS			
three-cracker assortment	4	13	100
Tiny Goldfish See SNACKS			
Pillsbury			
bread sticks See BREADS, ROLLS, BISCUITS, & MUFFINS			
Quaker Oats			
rice cakes, lightly salted, plain, multigrain, or sesame	1	7	35
Rokeach			
saltines	10	20	120
snack crackers	9	19	130
Sunshine			
American Heritage			
cheddar	5	8	80
sesame	4	8	70
Cheez-It	12	7	70
Hi Ho	4	8	80
Krispy saltines	5	11	60
oyster & soup	16	10	60
wheat wafers	8	10	80

❏ **CREAM & CREAM SUBSTITUTES**
See MILK, MILK SUBSTITUTES,
& MILK PRODUCTS

❏ **CROUTONS** *See* BREADCRUMBS,
CROUTONS, STUFFINGS, & SEASONED
COATINGS

❏ **CUSTARDS** *See* DESSERTS: CUSTARDS,
GELATINS, PUDDINGS, & PIE FILLINGS

	Portion	Carbohydrates (g)	Total Calories

ᴇLI MEATS *See* PROCESSED MEAT & POULTRY PRODUCTS

DESSERTS: CAKES, PASTRIES, & PIES

Cake & Coffee Cake

	Portion	Carbohydrates (g)	Total Calories
angel food			
from mix	whole (9¾" diam tube)	342	1,510
	¹⁄₁₂ cake	29	125
homemade	2.1 oz	36	161
applesauce spice, from mix	¹⁄₁₂ cake	34	250
banana, from mix	¹⁄₁₂ cake	36	260
w/buttercream icing	1.8 oz	29	181
Boston cream pie	3.9 oz	55	332
butter brickle, from mix	¹⁄₁₂ cake	37	260
butter pecan, from mix	¹⁄₁₂ cake	35	250
	⅛ cake	39	310
caramel, from mix	1.6 oz	24	173
w/caramel icing	1.9 oz	33	208
carrot			
from mix	¹⁄₁₂ cake	35	250
homemade, w/cream cheese icing	whole (10" diam tube)	775	6,175
	¹⁄₁₆ cake	48	385
cheesecake			
commercial	whole (9" diam)	317	3,350
	¹⁄₁₂ cake	26	280
from mix	⅛ cake	38	300
cherry chip, from mix	¹⁄₁₂ cake	36	180
chocolate	¹⁄₁₂ cake	35	250
w/icing, from mix	1.3 oz cup-cake	21	129
chocolate chip, from mix	¹⁄₁₂ cake	35	190
chocolate fudge bundt ring, from mix	¹⁄₁₆ cake	37	270
chocolate fudge w/vanilla icing, from mix	⅙ cake	46	280
chocolate macaroon bundt ring, from mix	¹⁄₁₆ cake	35	250
chocolate mint, from mix	¹⁄₁₂ cake	33	250
chocolate pudding, from mix	⅙ cake	45	230
cinnamon streusel, from mix	⅛ cake	41	250
coffee cake, crumb, from mix	whole = 15.1 oz	225	1,385
	⅙ cake	38	230

	Portion	Carbohydrates (g)	C...
cottage pudding, homemade	1.8 oz	27	1...
w/chocolate sauce	2½ oz	40	22...
w/fruit sauce	2½ oz	34	204
devil's food, homemade	2.1 oz	30	227
devil's food, w/chocolate icing			
from mix, made w/margarine	whole, 2-layer (8″ or 9″ diam)	645	3,755
	¹⁄₁₆ cake	40	235
	1.2 oz cup-cake	20	120
homemade	2.1 oz	34	233
fruitcake			
dark, homemade	3 lbs	783	5,185
	1½ oz	25	165
light	1.4 oz	23	156
German chocolate, from mix	¹⁄₁₂ cake	36	260
gingerbread			
from mix	whole (8″ square)	291	1,575
	⅑ cake	32	175
homemade	2½ oz	35	267
lemon, from mix	¹⁄₁₂ cake	36	260
lemon bundt ring, from mix	¹⁄₁₆ cake	43	270
lemon chiffon, from mix	¹⁄₁₂ cake	35	190
lemon pudding, from mix	⅙ cake	45	230
marble, from mix	¹⁄₁₂ cake	40	270
w/white icing	1.8 oz	31	165
marble streusel, w/icing, from mix	2.3 oz	33	224
orange			
from mix	¹⁄₁₂ cake	36	260
homemade, w/icing	1.8 oz	30	183
pineapple upside-down			
from mix	⅑ cake	43	270
homemade	2.6 oz	37	236
plum pudding, canned	3.6 oz	61	270
pound			
commercial	1.1 lb loaf	257	1,935
	1 oz	15	110
from mix	¹⁄₁₂ cake	27	200
homemade	1.1 lb	265	2,025
	1 oz	15	120
sheet, plain, homemade, w/ vegetable oil			
unfrosted	whole (9″ square)	434	2,830
	⅑ cake	48	315
w/uncooked white icing	whole (9″ square)	694	4,020
	⅑ cake	77	445

	Portion	Carbohydrates (g)	Total Calories
cake	0.9 oz	12	86
blackberries	5.2 oz	58	347
w/peaches	5.3 oz	42	266
w/raspberries	5.6 oz	47	290
w/strawberries	6.2 oz	61	344
snack cake, small, commercial			
devil's food w/cream filling	1 oz	17	105
sponge w/cream filling	1½ oz	27	155
sour cream, from mix	⅛ cake	35	270
chocolate	1/12 cake	36	260
white	1/12 cake	36	180
spice, from mix	1.8 oz	28	175
w/vanilla icing	1.8 oz	30	176
sponge, homemade	2.3 oz	36	188
w/strawberries & whipped cream	5.4 oz	60	328
strawberry, from mix	1/12 cake	36	260
streusel swirl, from mix	1/16 cake	38	260
white			
from mix	2½ oz	31	219
homemade	2.7 oz	41	285
white, w/chocolate icing, homemade	2.7 oz	46	298
white, w/white icing, commercial	whole, 2-layer (8″ or 9″ diam)	670	4,170
	1/16 cake	42	260
yellow, homemade	2.6 oz	39	283
yellow, w/chocolate icing			
commercial	whole, 2-layer (8″ or 9″ diam)	620	3,895
	1/16 cake	39	245
from mix	whole, 2-layer (8″ or 9″ diam)	638	3,735
	1/16 cake	40	235
homemade	2.6 oz	44	292
yellow cupcake			
w/chocolate icing	1.4 oz	25	155
w/vanilla icing	1.4 oz	25	160

Cake Icing

caramel	1.4 oz	24	140
chocolate	1.4 oz	26	148
chocolate, double dark	1.3 oz	26	150
chocolate fudge	1.4 oz	27	150
coconut	1.4 oz	29	140
coconut almond	1.2 oz	17	170
coconut pecan	1.2 oz	20	150

	Portion	Carbohydrates (g)	C
lemon	1.2 oz	25	l
milk chocolate	1.1 oz	26	15
strawberry	1.1 oz	25	140
vanilla	1.3 oz	25	150
white, fluffy	0.6 oz	17	70

Danish, Doughnuts, Sweet Rolls, & Toaster Pastries

danish pastry			
plain, w/out fruit or nuts	12 oz ring	152	1,305
	1 (4¼″ diam)	26	220
	1 oz	13	110
cinnamon raisin, from refrigerator dough	2.7 oz	40	270
fruit	1 round	28	235
doughnuts			
cake type, plain	1.8 oz	24	210
yeast-leavened, glazed	2.1 oz	26	235
sweet roll	1	21	154
cinnamon w/icing, from refrigerator dough	2	35	230
toaster pastries	1	38	210

Fruit Bettys, Cobblers, Crisps, & Turnovers

apple brown Betty	½ c	42	211
apple crisp	½ c	58	302
apple dumpling	1	31	280
cherry crisp	½ c	55	226
peach cobbler	⅓ c	25	160
peach crisp	½ c	37	249
turnover, from mix, apple, blueberry, or cherry	1	23	173

Pastry

cream puff, w/custard filling	3.7 oz	22	245
éclair			
w/chocolate icing & custard filling	3.9 oz	39	316
frozen	2 oz	27	205
w/chocolate icing & whipped cream filling	3.7 oz	15	296
lady finger, w/whipped cream filling	4 oz	38	326

pastry shells & pie crusts *See* BAKING INGREDIENTS

	Portion	Carbohydrates (g)	Total Calories
e, w/vegetable shortening crust	whole (9″ diam)	360	2,420
	⅙ pie	60	405
anana custard, homemade	5.6 oz	49	353
blackberry, homemade	5.6 oz	55	389
blueberry, w/vegetable shortening crust	whole (9″ diam)	330	2,285
	⅙ pie	55	380
butterscotch, homemade	5.6 oz	61	427
cherry, w/vegetable shortening crust	whole (9″ diam)	363	2,465
	⅙ pie	61	410
chocolate chiffon, homemade	2.8 oz	35	262
chocolate cream, homemade	4 oz	34	301
coconut custard, homemade	5½ oz	39	365
cream, w/vegetable shortening crust	whole (9″ diam)	351	2,710
	⅙ pie	59	455
custard, w/vegetable shortening crust	whole (9″ diam)	213	1,985
	⅙ pie	36	330
fried			
apple	3 oz	31	255
cherry	3 oz	32	250
lemon chiffon, homemade	3.8 oz	45	288
lemon meringue, w/vegetable shortening crust	whole (9″ diam)	317	2,140
	⅙ pie	53	355
mincemeat, homemade	5.6 oz	60	434
peach, w/vegetable shortening crust	whole (9″ diam)	361	2,410
	⅙ pie	60	405
pecan, w/vegetable shortening crust	whole (9″ diam)	423	3,450
	⅙ pie	71	575
pineapple cheese, homemade	5.6 oz piece	40	270
pumpkin, w/vegetable shortening crust	whole (9″ diam)	223	1,920
	⅙ pie	37	320
raisin, homemade	4.2 oz	52	325
rhubarb, homemade	5.6 oz	61	405
shoofly, homemade	3.9 oz	71	441
strawberry, homemade	4 oz	36	228
sweet potato, homemade	5.6 oz	38	342

Pie Fillings *See* DESSERTS: CUSTARDS, GELATINS, PUDDINGS, & PIE FILLINGS

	Portion	Carbohydrates (g)	Total Calories
• **BRAND NAME**			
Dromedary			
date nut roll	½″ slice	13	80
Kellogg's			
FROSTED POP-TARTS			
blueberry	1	38	200
brown sugar cinnamon	1	34	210
chocolate fudge	1	36	200
Dutch apple	1	36	210
peanut butter & jelly	1	34	220
POP-TARTS			
blueberry	1	36	210
brown sugar cinnamon	1	33	210
Nabisco			
Frosted Toastettes or Toastettes, all flavors	1	36	200
Pepperidge Farm Frozen Cakes & Pastries			
FRUIT SQUARES			
apple	1	27	220
blueberry	1	28	220
cherry	1	28	230
LAYER CAKES			
coconut	1⅝ oz	24	180
devil's food	1⅝ oz	24	170
German chocolate	1⅝ oz	22	180
golden	1⅝ oz	24	180
vanilla	1⅝ oz	24	170
OLD FASHIONED CAKES			
butter pound	1 oz	15	120
carrot w/cream cheese icing	1⅜ oz	16	130
PUFF PASTRY			
apple dumplings	3 oz	33	260
apple strudel	3 oz	35	240
patty shells	1	16	210
puff pastry sheets	¼ sheet	22	260
turnovers			
apple	1	34	300
blueberry	1	32	310
cherry	1	32	310
peach	1	34	310
raspberry	1	36	310

	Portion	Carbohydrates (g)	Total Calories
SUPREME CAKES			
Boston cream	2⅞ oz	39	290
chocolate	2⅞ oz	37	300
Grand Marnier	1½ oz	22	160
lemon coconut	3 oz	38	280
raspberry mocha	3⅛ oz	43	310
strawberry cream	2 oz	30	190
Pillsbury			
SWEET ROLLS			
Best apple danish w/icing	1	33	240
Best Quick cinnamon rolls w/ icing	1	29	210
cinnamon raisin danish w/icing	2	39	290
cinnamon rolls w/icing	2	34	230
TURNOVERS			
apple	1	23	170
blueberry	1	22	170
cherry	1	24	170
Rich's			
Bavarian cream puffs	1	17	146
chocolate éclairs	2 oz	27	205
Sara Lee			
ALL BUTTER COFFEE CAKES			
butter streusel	⅛ cake	20	160
cheese	⅛ cake	23	210
pecan	⅛ cake	19	160
ALL BUTTER POUND CAKES			
Original	⅒ cake	14	130
Family Size	1/15 cake	14	130
chocolate chip	⅒ cake	19	130
walnut raisin	⅒ cake	20	140
ELEGANT ENDINGS			
Classic	⅙ pkg	29	350
INDIVIDUAL DANISH			
apple	1	15	120
cheese	1	13	130
cinnamon raisin	1	17	150
raspberry	1	18	130
LE PASTRIE CROISSANTS			
apple	1	36	260
chocolate	1	34	320
cinnamon-nut-raisin	1	44	350
strawberry	1	38	270

	Portion	Carbohydrates (g)	Total Calories
LIGHT CLASSICS			
French cheesecake			
plain	¹⁄₁₀ pkg	19	200
strawberry	¹⁄₁₀ pkg	22	200
mousse cake			
chocolate	¹⁄₁₀ pkg	18	200
strawberry	¹⁄₁₀ pkg	18	180
SINGLE-LAYER ICED CAKES			
banana	⅛ cake	28	170
carrot	⅛ cake	31	260
TWO-LAYER CAKES			
Black Forest	⅛ cake	28	190
strawberry shortcake	⅛ cake	26	190

❏ DESSERTS: CUSTARDS, GELATINS, PUDDINGS, & PIE FILLINGS

Custard

	Portion	Carbohydrates (g)	Total Calories
plain			
baked, homemade	½ c	15	153
boiled, homemade	½ c	18	164
from mix	½ c	23	161
banana	½ c	20	143
chocolate	½ c	20	142
coconut	½ c	20	144
lemon	½ c	20	143
vanilla	½ c	20	143

Gelatin

	Portion	Carbohydrates (g)	Total Calories
dry	1 envelope	0	25
made w/water, all flavors	½ c	19	81

Pudding

	Portion	Carbohydrates (g)	Total Calories
butterscotch, homemade	½ c	38	207
chocolate			
canned	5 oz	30	205
from mix, prepared w/whole milk			
regular	½ c	25	150
instant	½ c	27	155
homemade	½ c	37	219
Indian, baked, homemade	⅔ c	23	161
lemon snow, homemade	½ c	27	114

	Portion	Carbohydrates (g)	Total Calories
rice, from mix, prepared w/ whole milk	½ c	27	155
rice w/raisins, homemade	¾ c	39	212
tapioca			
canned	5 oz	28	160
from mix, prepared w/whole milk	½ c	25	145
homemade	½ c	17	133
vanilla			
canned	5 oz	33	220
from mix, prepared w/whole milk			
regular	½ c	25	145
instant	½ c	27	150
homemade	½ c	24	152

Rennin Dessert

plain, homemade	½ c	15	113
chocolate, from mix			
prepared w/whole milk	½ c	17	127
prepared w/skim milk	½ c	18	95
fruit vanilla, from mix			
prepared w/whole milk	½ c	19	140
prepared w/skim milk	½ c	17	88

▪ BRAND NAME

D-Zerta

gelatin, low-cal	½ c	0	8
pudding, reduced-calorie, prepared w/skim milk			
chocolate	½ c	11	60
vanilla	½ c	12	70

Featherweight

custard, lemon or vanilla	½ c	8	40
gelatin, low-sodium, low-cal, all flavors	½ c	1	10
mousse, low-cal, chocolate	½ c	12	85
pudding: butterscotch, chocolate, or vanilla	½ c	3	12

Jell-O

AMERICANA DESSERTS, PREPARED W/WHOLE MILK

golden egg custard	½ c	23	160
rice pudding	½ c	30	170
tapioca pudding			
chocolate	½ c	28	170
vanilla	½ c	27	160

	Portion	Carbohydrates (g)	Total Calories
GELATIN			
average values, all flavors	½ c	19	80
PUDDING & PIE FILLING			
Regular, Prepared w/Whole Milk			
butterscotch	½ c	30	170
chocolate	½ c	28	160
vanilla	½ c	27	160
Instant, Prepared w/Whole Milk			
banana cream	½ c	28	160
butterscotch	½ c	28	160
chocolate	½ c	30	180
lemon	½ c	29	170
vanilla	½ c	29	170
Sugar-free, Prepared w/2% Low-Fat Milk			
chocolate	½ c	13	90
vanilla	½ c	11	80
Sugar-free Instant, Prepared w/2% Low-Fat Milk			
banana	½ c	13	90
butterscotch	½ c	13	90
chocolate	½ c	14	100
vanilla	½ c	13	90
RICH & DELICIOUS MOUSSE, PREPARED W/WHOLE MILK			
chocolate or chocolate fudge	½ c	21	150
Rich's Puddings			
butterscotch	3 oz	18	133
chocolate	3 oz	18	141
vanilla	3 oz	18	129
Royal			
GELATIN			
all flavors			
regular	½ c	19	80
sugar-free	½ c	0	6
PUDDING & PIE FILLING			
Cooked			
banana cream, prepared	½ c	27	160
butterscotch, prepared	½ c	27	160
chocolate			
dry	0.9 oz	25	120
prepared	½ c	33	180
custard, prepared	½ c	22	150
Dark 'n Sweet, prepared	½ c	33	180

	Portion	Carbohydrates (g)	Total Calories
flan w/caramel sauce, prepared	½ c	22	150
key lime, prepared	½ c	30	160
lemon			
dry	½ oz	13	50
prepared	½ c	30	160
vanilla			
dry	0.7 oz	20	80
prepared	½ c	27	160
Instant			
banana cream, prepared	½ c	29	180
butterscotch, prepared	½ c	29	180
chocolate			
dry	1 oz	25	120
prepared	½ c	35	190
Dark 'n Sweet, prepared	½ c	35	190
lemon			
dry	0.8 oz	24	110
prepared	½ c	29	180
pistachio nut, prepared	½ c	30	170
vanilla			
dry	0.8 oz	24	100
prepared	½ c	29	180
Instant Sugar-free			
butterscotch, prepared	½ c	16	100
chocolate			
dry	½ oz	11	50
prepared	½ c	17	110
vanilla			
dry	0.4 oz	10	40
prepared	½ c	16	100

❑ DESSERTS, FROZEN: ICE CREAM, ICE MILK, ICES & SHERBETS, & FROZEN JUICE, PUDDING, TOFU, & YOGURT

Frozen Pudding on a Stick

banana	1	16	94
butterscotch	1	16	94
chocolate	1	17	99
chocolate fudge	1	17	99
vanilla	1	16	93

	Portion	Carbohydrates (g)	Total Calories

Frozen Yogurt

IN A CUP

fruit varieties	½ c	21	108

ON A STICK

plain	1	13	65
carob/chocolate-coated	1	13	135
raspberry, chocolate-coated	1	15	127
strawberry	1	13	69

Ice Cream

chocolate	1 c	33	295
French custard	1 c	28	257
French vanilla, soft serve	1 c	38	377
strawberry	1 c	31	250
vanilla			
10% fat	1 c	32	269
16% fat	1 c	32	349

Ice Cream Novelties & Cones

ice cream cone (cone only)	1	9	45
ice cream sandwich	1	26	167
vanilla ice cream bar w/chocolate coating	1	15	162
vanilla ice milk bar w/chocolate coating	1	16	144

Ice Milk

chocolate	⅔ c	20	137
strawberry	⅔ c	22	133
vanilla			
regular	1 c	29	184
soft serve	1 c	38	223

Ices & Sherbets

lemon sherbet	¾ c	45	241
lime/orange ice	1 c	63	247
	⅔ c	42	165
orange sherbet	1 c	59	270
sherbet, various flavors	1 c	58	236

	Portion	Carbohydrates (g)	Total Calories

- **BRAND NAME**

Baskin-Robbins
CONES

cake	1	4	19
sugar	1	11	57

ICE CREAM & SHERBET

chocolate	4 oz	33	264
Chocolate Mousse Royale	4 oz	36	293
French vanilla	4 oz	25	290
orange sherbet	4 oz	33	158
Pralines 'n Cream	4 oz	38	283
raspberry sorbet	4 oz	34	134
Rocky Road	4 oz	43	291
strawberry	4 oz	25	226
vanilla	4 oz	25	235
wild strawberry (low-fat)	4 oz	25	90

Comet

cups	1	4	20
sugar cones	1	9	40

Dole
FRUIT & CREAM BARS

blueberry, peach, or strawberry	1	19	90

FRUIT 'N JUICE BARS

banana	1	20	80
orange w/mandarin	1	18	70
piña colada	1	16	90
pineapple	1	17	70
raspberry	1	16	70
strawberry	1	16	70

SORBETS

mandarin orange	4 oz	28	110
peach	4 oz	28	120
pineapple	4 oz	28	120
raspberry	4 oz	28	110
strawberry	4 oz	28	110

Drumstick

Drumstick sundae cone	1	22	186

Jell-O
FRUIT BARS

all flavors	1	11	45

GELATIN POPS

all flavors	1	8	35

	Portion	Carbohydrates (g)	Total Calories
PUDDING POPS			
chocolate	1	13	80
chocolate-covered vanilla	1	14	130
vanilla w/chocolate chips	1	13	80
Land O'Lakes			
ice cream, vanilla	4 fl oz	16	140
ice milk, vanilla	4 fl oz	14	90
sherbet, fruit flavors	4 fl oz	27	130
Life Savers			
Flavor Pops, all flavors	1	10	40
Minute Maid Frozen Fruit Juice Bars			
cherry, fruit punch, grape, orange, strawberry (Variety Pack)	2¼ oz	14	60
Oreo Cookies 'n Cream *ICE CREAM*			
chocolate	3 fl oz	16	140
vanilla	3 fl oz	16	140
NOVELTIES			
on a stick	1	19	220
sandwich	1	31	240
Snackwich	1	8	60
Popsicle			
Creamsicle	1	18	103
Fudgsicle	1	19	91
Popsicle	1	17	65
Tofutti *LITE LITE*			
all flavors	4 oz	20	90
PINTS			
Cappuccino Love Drops	4 fl oz	26	230
Chocolate Love Drops	4 fl oz	26	230
Chocolate Supreme	4 fl oz	20	210
vanilla	4 fl oz	21	200
vanilla almond bark	4 fl oz	23	230
Vanilla Love Drops	4 fl oz	26	220
wildberry	4 fl oz	22	210
SINGLE SERVINGS			
Chocolate Cuties	1	21	140
Vanilla Cuties	1	21	130
SOFT SERVE			
regular	4 fl oz	20	158
Hi-Lite			
chocolate	4 fl oz	18	100
vanilla	4 fl oz	18	90

	Portion	Carbohydrates (g)	Total Calories

DESSERT SAUCES, SYRUPS, & TOPPINGS

See also NUTS & NUT-BASED BUTTERS, FLOURS, MEALS, MILKS, PASTES, & POWDERS

Sauces, Syrups, & Flavored Toppings

	Portion	Carbohydrates (g)	Total Calories
butterscotch sauce, homemade	2 T	40	203
butterscotch topping	3 T	39	156
caramel topping	3 T	39	155
cherry topping	3 T	38	147
chocolate-flavored syrup or topping			
fudge type	2 T	21	125
thin type	2 T	22	85
custard sauce, homemade	4 T	9	85
hard sauce, homemade	4 T	24	193
honey *See* SUGARS & SWEETENERS			
lemon sauce, homemade	4 T	29	133
pineapple topping	3 T	37	146
walnuts in syrup topping	3 T	38	169

Whipped Cream & Whipped Cream–Type Toppings

	Portion	Carbohydrates (g)	Total Calories
nondairy			
powdered, prepared w/whole	1 T	1	8
milk	1 c	13	151
pressurized, containing lauric	1 T	1	11
acid oil & sodium caseinate	1 c	11	184
semisolid, frozen, containing	1 T	1	13
lauric acid oil & sodium caseinate	1 c	17	239
whipped cream topping, pressurized	1 T	tr	8
surized	1 c	7	154

▪ BRAND NAME

Cool Whip

	Portion	Carbohydrates (g)	Total Calories
Extra Creamy Dairy Recipe whipped topping	1 T	1	16
nondairy whipped topping	1 T	1	12

Dream Whip

	Portion	Carbohydrates (g)	Total Calories
whipped topping mix, prepared w/whole milk	1 T	1	10

	Portion	Carbohydrates (g)	Total Calories
D-Zerta			
reduced-calorie whipped topping	1 T	0	8
Featherweight			
whipped topping	1 T	0	2
Hershey			
chocolate fudge topping	2 T	14	100
Smucker's			
butterscotch	2 T	33	140
caramel	2 T	33	140
chocolate fudge	2 T	31	130
fruit syrups	2 T	26	100
hot caramel	2 T	28	150
hot fudge	2 T	18	110
peanut butter caramel	2 T	29	150
pineapple	2 T	32	130
strawberry	2 T	30	120
walnuts in syrup	2 T	27	130

❑ DINNERS, FROZEN

• BRAND NAME

	Portion	Carbohydrates (g)	Total Calories
Health Valley Lean Living			
cheese enchiladas	9 oz	43	280
chicken à la king	9 oz	30	380
chicken crêpes	9 oz	23	380
spinach lasagna	9 oz	26	170
Hungry-Man Dinners See Swanson, below			
Lean Cuisine See Stouffer, below			
Le Menu			
beef sirloin tips	11½ oz	29	410
beef Stroganoff	10 oz	28	450
breast of chicken parmigiana	11½ oz	29	390
chicken à la king	10¼ oz	30	330
chicken cordon bleu	11 oz	49	470
chicken Florentine	12½ oz	39	480
chopped sirloin beef	12¼ oz	36	410
ham steak	10 oz	35	310
pepper steak	11½ oz	37	380
sliced breast of turkey w/mushrooms	11¼ oz	36	460

	Portion	Carbohydrates (g)	Total Calories
stuffed flounder	10¼ oz	28	350
sweet & sour chicken	11¼ oz	42	460
vegetable lasagna	11 oz	33	360
Yankee pot roast	11 oz	29	360
Le Menu Light Style			
beef à l'orange	10 oz	31	290
chicken cacciatore	10 oz	22	260
flounder vin blanc	10 oz	26	220
glazed chicken breast	10 oz	28	240
3-cheese stuffed shells	10 oz	37	280
turkey divan	10 oz	21	280
L'Orient			
beef broccoli	11 oz	34	530
Cantonese chicken chow mein	11½ oz	34	280
Firecracker chicken	10½ oz	41	380
lemon chicken	11 oz	43	400
orange beef	10¾ oz	42	380
rock sugar–glazed pork	10¾ oz	29	360
Stouffer			
DINNER SUPREME			
baked chicken breast w/gravy	11 oz	31	330
beef teriyaki	11⅜ oz	34	370
beef tips Bourguignonne	12⅜ oz	22	360
chicken Florentine	11 oz	32	430
chicken w/Supreme Sauce	11⅜ oz	29	360
flounder w/dill cream sauce	11⅝ oz	27	370
flounder w/roasted red pepper sauce	12 oz	27	360
Salisbury steak w/gravy & mushrooms	13½ oz	28	380
LEAN CUISINE			
beef & pork cannelloni w/Mornay sauce	9⅝ oz	25	270
breast of chicken Marsala w/vegetables	8⅛ oz	11	190
cheese cannelloni w/tomato sauce	9⅛ oz	24	270
chicken à l'orange w/almond rice	8 oz	31	270
chicken & vegetables w/vermicelli	12¾ oz	29	270
chicken cacciatore w/vermicelli	10⅞ oz	25	280
chicken chow mein w/rice	11¼ oz	36	250
filet of fish divan	12⅜ oz	17	270
filet of fish Florentine	9 oz	13	240
filet of fish jardiniere w/souffléed potatoes	11¼ oz	18	280
glazed chicken w/vegetable rice	8½ oz	23	270
herbed lamb w/rice	10⅜ oz	29	280

	Portion	Carbohydrates (g)	Total Calories
linguini w/clam sauce	9⅝ oz	32	260
meatball stew	10 oz	20	250
Oriental beef w/vegetables & rice	8⅝ oz	30	270
Oriental scallops & vegetables w/rice	11 oz	34	220
Salisbury steak w/Italian-style sauce & vegetables	9½ oz	14	270
shrimp & chicken Cantonese w/noodles	10⅛ oz	22	270
spaghetti w/beef & mushroom sauce	11½ oz	38	280
stuffed cabbage w/meat in to-mato sauce	10¾ oz	20	220
tuna lasagna w/spinach noo-dles & vegetables	9¾ oz	28	280
turkey Dijon	9½ oz	21	280
veal lasagna	10¼ oz	24	280
veal primavera	9⅛ oz	19	250
zucchini lasagna	11 oz	28	260
Swanson			
3-COMPARTMENT DINNERS			
beans & franks	10½ oz	55	420
macaroni & beef	12 oz	48	370
macaroni & cheese	12¼ oz	48	380
noodles & chicken	10½ oz	37	270
spaghetti & meatballs	12½ oz	46	370
4-COMPARTMENT DINNERS			
beans & franks	10½ oz	66	500
beef	11¼ oz	41	350
beef enchiladas	13¾ oz	52	480
beef in barbecue sauce	11 oz	49	460
chicken in barbecue sauce	11¾ oz	53	450
chicken nugget platter	8¾ oz	40	470
chopped sirloin beef	11 oz	29	380
fish & chips	10 oz	62	500
fish nugget	9½ oz	44	450
fried chicken			
barbecue-flavored	edible portion = 10 oz	56	580
dark meat	edible portion = 10 oz	58	580
white meat	edible portion = 10½ oz	62	580
loin of pork	10¾ oz	26	310
meat loaf	10¾ oz	41	430
Mexican-style combination	14¼ oz	54	500
Polynesian style	12 oz	52	360
Salisbury steak	10¾ oz	43	410

	Portion	Carbohydrates (g)	Total Calories
sweet & sour chicken	12 oz	48	390
Swiss steak	10 oz	37	350
turkey	11½ oz	43	360
veal parmigiana	12¼ oz	42	460
Western style	11½ oz	42	440
HUNGRY-MAN DINNERS			
boneless chicken	17¾ oz	68	710
chicken nuggets	16 oz	69	600
chicken parmigiana	20 oz	53	810
chopped beef steak	16¾ oz	46	590
fish & chips	14¾ oz	73	780
fried chicken			
breast portions	14½ oz	83	930
dark portions	edible portion = 14½ oz	81	910
lasagna	18¾ oz	100	740
Mexican style	20¼ oz	75	750
Salisbury steak	18¼ oz	32	660
sliced beef	15½ oz	50	470
turkey	17 oz	61	550
veal parmigiana	18¼ oz	61	630
Western style	17½ oz	66	740

❏ EGGS & EGG SUBSTITUTES

Chicken Eggs

COOKED

egg dishes, prepared *See* BREAKFAST FOODS, PREPARED; FAST FOODS

	Portion	Carbohydrates (g)	Total Calories
fried in butter	1 large	1	83
hard boiled	1 large	1	79
omelet, cooked w/butter & milk	1 egg (large)	1	95
poached	1 large	1	79
scrambled, w/butter & milk	1 large	1	95

DRIED

	Portion	Carbohydrates (g)	Total Calories
whole	1 c sifted	4	505
whole, stabilized (glucose-reduced)	1 c sifted	2	523
white only			
flakes, stabilized (glucose-reduced)	½ lb	9	796
powder, stabilized (glucose-reduced)	1 c sifted	5	402
yolk only	1 c sifted	tr	460

	Portion	Carbohydrates (g)	Total Calories
UNCOOKED			
whole, fresh or frozen	1	1	79
white only, fresh or frozen	1	0	16
yolk only, fresh	1	tr	63
Eggs, Other			
duck	1	1	130
goose	1	2	267
quail	1	tr	14
turkey	1	1	135
Egg Substitute			
frozen, containing egg white, corn oil, & nonfat dry milk	¼ c	2	96
liquid, containing egg white, soybean oil, & soy protein	1 c	2	211
powder, containing egg white solids, whole egg solids, sweet whey solids, nonfat dry milk, & soy protein	0.7 oz	4	88

• **BRAND NAME**

	Portion	Carbohydrates (g)	Total Calories
Featherweight			
egg substitute	2 eggs	2	120
Fleischmann's			
Egg Beaters	¼ c	1	25
Egg Beaters w/Cheez	½ c	3	130
Oregon Freeze Dry			
cheese omelet	2 eggs	11	240
eggs, w/butter	2 eggs	9	183
precooked eggs, w/real bacon	2 eggs	2	180

❑ **ENTREES & MAIN COURSES, CANNED & BOXED**

chili & bean products, canned & boxed *See* LEGUMES & LEGUME PRODUCTS; SOYBEANS & SOYBEAN PRODUCTS

	Portion	Carbohydrates (g)	Total Calories

- **BRAND NAME**

Armour Star

beef stew	7½ oz	16	210

corned roast beef hash & sloppy joes *See* PROCESSED MEAT & POULTRY
   PRODUCTS

Chun King
DIVIDER PAK ENTREES, CANNED

4 Servings/42 Oz Pkg

beef chow mein	7 oz	12	100
beef pepper Oriental	7 oz	11	110
chicken chow mein	7 oz	11	110
pork chow mein	7 oz	11	120
shrimp chow mein	7 oz	13	100

2 Servings/24 Oz Pkg

beef chow mein	8 oz	13	110
chicken chow mein	8 oz	13	120

STIR-FRY ENTREES, CANNED

chow mein w/beef	6 oz	11	290
chow mein w/chicken	6 oz	11	220
egg foo young	5 oz	9	140
pepper steak	6 oz	9	250
sukiyaki	6 oz	10	260

Featherweight

beef ravioli	8 oz	33	220
beef stew	7½ oz	24	220
boned chicken	13 oz	0	186
chicken stew	7½ oz	21	170
chicken w/dumplings	7½ oz	18	160
spaghetti w/meatballs	7½ oz	28	200

Franco-American

beef ravioli in meat sauce	7½ oz	36	230
macaroni & cheese	7⅜ oz	24	170
PizzO's	7½ oz	35	170
spaghetti in tomato sauce w/ cheese	7⅜ oz	36	190
SpaghettiO's in tomato & cheese sauce	7⅜ oz	34	170
spaghetti w/meatballs in to- mato sauce	7⅜ oz	28	220

Noodle-Roni Pasta

chicken & mushroom flavor, prepared	½ c	25	150
fettucini, prepared	½ c	29	300
garlic & butter, prepared	½ c	29	290
herbs & butter, prepared	½ c	19	160

	Portion	Carbohydrates (g)	Total Calories
parmesano, prepared	½ c	23	230
pesto Italiano, prepared	½ c	23	210
Rominoff, prepared	½ c	28	240
Stroganoff, prepared	¾ c	36	360
Swanson			
chicken à la king	5¼ oz	9	180
chicken & dumplings	7½ oz	19	220
chicken stew	7⅝ oz	16	170
Van Camp's			
Noodle Weenee	1 c	33	245
tamales w/sauce	1 c	29	293

❑ ENTREES & MAIN COURSES, FROZEN

	Portion	Carbohydrates (g)	Total Calories
Celentano			
baked pasta & cheese	12 oz	60	530
broccoli stuffed shells	11½ oz	46	400
cannelloni Florentine	12 oz	36	380
cavatelli	3.2 oz	57	270
chicken cutlets parmigiana	9 oz	40	310
chicken primavera	11½ oz	15	270
eggplant parmigiana	8 oz	22	330
	7 oz	32	270
Eggplant Rollettes	11 oz	18	420
lasagne	8 oz	30	320
	6¼ oz	58	250
lasagne primavera	11 oz	36	300
manicotti			
w/sauce	8 oz	22	300
w/out sauce	7 oz	34	380
ravioli			
miniround cheese, w/out sauce	4 oz	37	250
round cheese, w/out sauce	6½ oz	51	410
stuffed shells			
w/sauce	8 oz	30	320
w/out sauce	6¼ oz	33	350
Lean Cuisine See Stouffer, *under* DINNERS, FROZEN			
Le Menu Entrees			
beef burgundy	7½ oz	5	330
chicken Kiev	8 oz	24	530
manicotti	8½ oz	27	300
Oriental chicken	8½ oz	31	260
Mrs. Paul's			
eggplant parmigiana See VEGETABLES, PLAIN & PREPARED			

	Portion	Carbohydrates (g)	Total Calories
AU NATUREL SEAFOOD			
cod fillets	4 oz	0	90
flounder fillets	4 oz	0	90
haddock fillets	4 oz	0	80
perch fillets	4 oz	0	80
sole fillets	4 oz	0	90
BUTTERED SEAFOOD			
fish fillets	2	4	170
LIGHT SEAFOOD ENTREES			
fish & pasta Florentine	9½ oz	19	240
fish au gratin	10 oz	23	290
fish Dijon	9½ oz	11	280
fish Florentine	9 oz	13	210
fish Mornay	10 oz	17	280
shrimp & clams w/linguini	10 oz	43	280
shrimp Cajun style	10½ oz	29	200
shrimp Oriental	11 oz	46	280
shrimp primavera	11 oz	36	240
tuna pasta casserole	11 oz	32	290
PREPARED BATTERED SEAFOOD			
batter-dipped fish fillets	2	31	390
Crunchy Light Batter			
fish fillets	2	28	310
fish sticks	4	23	240
flounder fillets	2	29	310
haddock fillets	2	35	330
fried clams in a light batter	2½ oz	22	240
PREPARED BREADED SEAFOOD			
catfish fillets	1	20	220
combination seafood platter	9 oz	58	590
Crispy Crunchy			
fish fillets	2	26	280
fish sticks	4	19	200
flounder fillets	2	23	270
haddock fillets	2	21	250
perch fillets	2	25	320
deviled crabs	1 piece	21	190
fish cakes	2	27	250
french-fried scallops	3½ oz	26	230
fried shrimp	3 oz	16	200
Supreme Light Breaded			
fish fillets	1	21	290
flounder or sole fillets	1	19	280
Sara Lee Le Sandwich Croissants			
cheddar cheese	1	29	380
chicken & broccoli	1	32	340

	Portion	Carbohydrates (g)	Total Calories
ham & Swiss cheese	1	30	340
turkey, bacon, & cheese	1	30	370

Stouffer
ENTREES

	Portion	Carbohydrates (g)	Total Calories
beef & spinach stuffed pasta shells w/tomato sauce	9 oz	27	300
beef chop suey w/rice	12 oz	38	340
beef pie	10 oz	36	560
beef stew	10 oz	19	310
beef Stroganoff w/parsley noodles	9¾ oz	29	410
beef teriyaki in sauce w/rice & vegetables	9¾ oz	35	330
cashew chicken in sauce w/ rice	9½ oz	33	410
cheese soufflé	7⅝ oz	16	480
cheese stuffed pasta shells w/ meat sauce	9 oz	25	340
chicken à la king w/rice	9½ oz	37	320
chicken chow mein w/out noodles	8 oz	11	140
chicken crêpes w/mushroom sauce	8¼ oz	18	370
chicken divan	8½ oz	14	350
chicken paprikash w/egg noodles	10½ oz	31	390
chicken pie	10 oz	34	530
chicken stuffed pasta shells w/ cheese sauce	9 oz	21	420
chili con carne w/beans	8¾ oz	23	280
creamed chicken	6½ oz	7	320
creamed chipped beef	5½ oz	8	240
escalloped chicken & noodles	5¾ oz	16	260
fettucini Alfredo	5 oz	17	280
fettucini primavera	½ of 10⅝ oz pkg	12	270
green pepper steak w/rice	10½ oz	38	340
Ham & Asparagus Bake	9½ oz	31	510
ham & asparagus crêpes	6¼ oz	24	310
ham & Swiss cheese crêpes w/ cream sauce	7½ oz	21	410
lasagna	10½ oz	34	370
linguini w/pesto sauce	½ of 8¼ oz pkg	20	210
lobster Newburg	6½ oz	8	360
macaroni & beef w/tomatoes	11½ oz	32	360
macaroni & cheese	6 oz	24	250
noodles Romanoff	4 oz	15	170
roast beef hash	5¾ oz	11	250
Salisbury steaks w/onion gravy	6 oz	6	230

	Portion	Carbohydrates (g)	Total Calories
Scallops & Shrimp Mariner w/ Rice	10¼ oz	35	390
short ribs of beef w/vegetable gravy	5¾ oz	2	280
spaghetti w/meatballs	12⅝ oz	43	370
spaghetti w/meat sauce	14 oz	53	440
spinach crêpes w/cheddar cheese sauce	9½ oz	27	420
steak & mushroom pie	10 oz	33	430
stuffed green peppers w/beef in tomato sauce	7¾ oz	18	220
Swedish meatballs in gravy w/ parsley noodles	11 oz	36	470
tuna noodle casserole	5¾ oz	18	190
turkey casserole w/gravy & dressing	9¾ oz	28	380
turkey pie	10 oz	36	540
turkey tetrazzini	6 oz	14	230
vegetable lasagna	10½ oz	29	450
Welsh rarebit	5 oz	9	360

LEAN CUISINE See Stouffer, *under* DINNERS, FROZEN

Swanson
CHICKEN DUET ENTREES

creamy broccoli	6 oz	18	310
creamy green bean	6 oz	20	330
saucy tomato	6 oz	21	340
savory wild rice	6 oz	22	290

CHICKEN DUET GOURMET NUGGETS

ham & cheese	3 oz	13	220
Mexican style	3 oz	14	220
pizza style	3 oz	15	210
spinach & herb	3 oz	15	230

CHUNKY PIES

beef	10 oz	53	550
chicken	10 oz	53	580
turkey	10 oz	46	540

DIPSTERS

barbecue	3 oz	13	220
Coconola	3 oz	12	240
herb	3 oz	12	220
Italian style	3 oz	8	230

ENTREES

Chicken Nibbles	edible portion = 5 oz	15	260
Fish 'n' Fries	7¼ oz	44	420

	Portion	Carbohydrates (g)	Total Calories
fried chicken	edible portion = 6½ oz	17	300
Salisbury steak	10 oz	9	410
Swedish meatballs	9¼ oz	16	420
turkey	8¾ oz	27	270
veal parmigiana	10 oz	22	280
HUNGRY-MAN POT PIES			
beef	16 oz	70	680
chicken	16 oz	65	730
turkey	16 oz	68	690
MAIN COURSE ENTREES			
lasagna w/meat	13¼ oz	51	470
macaroni & cheese	12 oz	47	390
PLUMP & JUICY			
chicken cutlets	3 oz	11	200
Chicken Dipsters	3 oz	12	220
Chicken Drumlets	3 oz	11	220
Chicken Nibbles	3¼ oz	16	300
Extra Crispy fried chicken	3 oz	15	250
fried chicken			
assorted pieces	3¼ oz	14	270
breast portions	4½ oz	20	360
Take-Out fried chicken, assorted pieces	3¼ oz	14	270
thighs & drumsticks	3¼ oz	12	280
POT PIES			
beef	8 oz	40	410
chicken	8 oz	33	420
macaroni & cheese	7 oz	27	220
turkey	8 oz	36	410
Tyson			
chicken cordon bleu	about 3½ oz	4	225
chicken Kiev	about 3½ oz	4	290
stuffed chicken breast	about 3½ oz	12	160

❑ FAST FOODS

shakes			
chocolate	10 fl oz	58	360
strawberry	10 fl oz	53	319
vanilla	10 fl oz	51	314
tacos	1	15	195

	Portion	Carbohydrates (g)	Total Calories

- ## BRAND NAME

Arby's
CHICKEN, ROASTED

	Portion	Carbohydrates (g)	Total Calories
breast	1	2	254
leg	1	1	319

DESSERTS

apple turnover	1	28	303
cherry turnover	1	25	280

SALADS

chicken salad & croissant	1	16	472
chicken salad w/tomato & lettuce	1	24	515
tossed salad			
plain	1	7	44
w/low-cal Italian dressing	1	9	57

SANDWICHES

Bac'n Cheddar Deluxe	1	33	526
Beef'n Cheddar	1	28	455
chicken breast	1	36	509
chicken club	1	57	621
chicken salad	1	33	386
fish fillet	1	51	580
hot ham & cheese	1	19	292
Philly Beef 'n Swiss	1	27	460
roast beef			
junior	1	22	218
regular	1	32	353
king	1	44	467
giant	1	46	531
super	1	50	501
Turkey Deluxe	1	33	375

SHAKES

chocolate	1	77	451
Jamocha	1	59	368
vanilla	1	46	330

SIDE DISHES

french fries	1 serving	30	215
potato cakes	1 serving	20	201
rice pilaf	1 serving	23	123
Scandinavian vegetables in sauce	1 serving	9	56

	Portion	Carbohydrates (g)	Total Calories
Burger King			
BREAKFAST ITEMS			
Breakfast Croissan'wich	1	20	304
w/bacon	1	20	355
w/ham	1	20	335
w/sausage	1	20	538
French toast sticks	1 serving	49	499
Great Danish	1	40	500
scrambled egg platter	1	33	468
w/bacon	1	33	536
w/sausage	1	33	702
BURGERS & SANDWICHES			
bacon double cheeseburger	1	27	510
cheeseburger	1	30	317
Chicken Specialty	1	56	688
Ham & Cheese Specialty	1	44	471
hamburger	1	29	275
Whaler fish	1	45	488
Whopper	1	46	628
w/cheese	1	47	711
Whopper Jr.	1	30	322
w/cheese	1	31	364
CHICKEN			
Chicken Tenders	6 pieces	10	204
DESSERTS			
apple pie	1 slice	44	305
SALADS			
plain salad	1 serving	5	28
w/bleu cheese dressing	1 serving	7	184
w/house dressing	1 serving	8	158
w/reduced-calorie Italian dressing	1 serving	7	42
w/Thousand Island dressing	1 serving	9	145
SHAKES			
chocolate	1 regular	46	320
syrup added	1 regular	60	374
vanilla	1 regular	49	321
syrup added	1 regular	51	334
SIDE DISHES			
french fries	1 regular serving	24	227
onion rings	1 regular serving	28	274

	Portion	Carbohydrates (g)	Total Calories
Church's Fried Chicken			
CHICKEN			
breast	1	9	278
leg	1	5	147
thigh	1	9	306
wing-breast	1 each	9	303
SIDE DISHES			
corn, w/butter oil	1 ear	33	237
french fries, w/salt	1 regular serving	20	138
Hardee's			
BREAKFAST ITEMS			
American cheese slice	1	2	47
bacon & egg biscuit	1	29	410
Big Country Breakfast bacon	1 serving	56	761
Big Country Breakfast ham	1 serving	51	665
Big Country Breakfast sausage	1 serving	23	849
biscuit gravy	1 serving	10	144
Canadian Sunrise biscuit	1	33	482
cinnamon & raisin biscuit	1	30	276
cheese biscuit	1	34	304
country ham biscuit	1	28	323
egg	1	1	79
egg biscuit	1	33	336
ham biscuit	1	31	300
Hash Rounds potatoes	1 serving	24	249
jam	1 serving	13	51
Rise 'n' Shine biscuit	1	32	257
sausage & egg biscuit	1	30	503
sausage biscuit	1	29	426
steak biscuit	1	46	491
BURGERS & SANDWICHES			
bacon cheeseburger	1	34	556
big deluxe burger	1	32	503
cheeseburger			
regular	1	32	327
¼ lb	1	35	511
chicken fillet	1	47	446
Fisherman's Fillet	1	47	469
hamburger	1	28	244
hot dog	1	28	285
hot ham & cheese	1	34	316
mushroom & Swiss burger	1	44	509
roast beef			
regular	1	30	312
big	1	35	440
turkey club	1	32	426

	Portion	Carbohydrates (g)	Total Calories
DESSERTS			
apple turnover	1	35	87
Big Cookie Treat	1	33	54
Cool Twist cone	1	26	164
SALADS			
chef salad	1	27	309
garden salad, w/Thousand Island dressing	1	37	501
side salad	1	21	90
SHAKES			
chocolate	1	63	390
SIDE DISHES			
french fries	1 regular serving	33	252
	1 large serving	54	438
Jack-in-the-Box			
BEVERAGES			
hot chocolate	1	24	133
BREAKFAST ITEMS			
Breakfast Jack	1	30	307
grape jelly	1 serving	9	38
pancake platter	1	87	612
pancake syrup	1 serving	30	121
scrambled egg platter	1	52	662
BURGERS & SANDWICHES			
bacon cheeseburger	1	48	705
cheeseburger	1	28	325
Chicken Supreme	1	34	575
club pita, w/out sauce	1	28	277
ham & Swiss burger	1	42	754
hamburger	1	29	288
Hot Club Supreme	1	38	524
Jumbo Jack	1	42	584
w/cheese	1	46	677
Moby Jack	1	39	444
Monterey burger	1	40	808
mushroom burger	1	41	513
Swiss & bacon burger	1	34	678
Ultimate Cheeseburger	1	33	942
CRESCENT ROLLS			
Canadian crescent	1	25	452
sausage crescent	1	28	584
Supreme crescent	1	27	547

	Portion	Carbohydrates (g)	Total Calories
DESSERTS			
cheesecake	1 piece	29	309
hot apple turnover	1	45	410
ENTREES			
chicken strip dinner	1	65	674
shrimp dinner	1	74	677
sirloin steak dinner	1	79	702
MEXICAN DISHES			
Fajita Pita	1	31	278
guacamole	1 serving	2	55
nachos			
cheese	1 serving	49	571
Supreme	1 serving	66	787
salsa	1 serving	2	8
taco	1	16	191
Super taco	1	21	288
PIZZA			
Pizza Pocket	1	42	497
SALAD DRESSINGS			
bleu cheese	1 serving	7	131
buttermilk house	1 serving	4	181
reduced-calorie French	1 serving	13	80
Thousand Island	1 serving	6	156
SALADS			
chef salad	1	3	295
pasta & seafood salad	1	32	394
side salad	1	<1	51
taco salad	1	10	377
SAUCES			
A-1 Steak	1 serving	5	18
BBQ	1 serving	10	39
Mayo-Mustard	1 serving	2	124
Mayo-Onion	1 serving	1	143
Seafood Cocktail	1 serving	12	57
SHAKES			
chocolate	1	55	330
strawberry	1	55	320
vanilla	1	57	320

	Portion	Carbohydrates (g)	Total Calories
SIDE DISHES			
french fries	1 regular serving	27	221
	1 large serving	43	353
onion rings	1 serving	39	382
Kentucky Fried Chicken			
FRIED CHICKEN			
Original Recipe			
breast			
center	1	8	257
side	1	10	276
drumstick	1	3	147
thigh	1	8	278
wing	1	6	181
Extra Crispy			
breast			
center	1	14	353
side	1	17	354
drumstick	1	6	173
thigh	1	14	371
wing	1	8	218
NUGGETS & SAUCES			
nuggets	1	2	46
barbecue sauce	1 oz	7	35
honey sauce	½ oz	12	49
mustard sauce	1 oz	6	36
sweet & sour sauce	1 oz	13	58
SIDE DISHES			
baked beans	1 serving	18	105
buttermilk biscuits	1	32	269
chicken gravy	1 serving	4	59
cole slaw	1 serving	12	103
corn on the cob	1 ear	32	176
Kentucky fries	1 serving	33	268
mashed potatoes	1 serving	12	59
w/gravy	1 serving	10	62
potato salad	1 serving	13	141
McDonald's			
BREAKFAST ITEMS			
biscuit			
w/bacon, cheese, & egg	1	33	483
w/biscuit spread	1	37	330
w/sausage	1	35	467
w/sausage & egg	1	36	585
danish			
apple	1	51	389

	Portion	Carbohydrates (g)	Total Calories
danish *(cont.)*			
cinnamon raisin	1	58	445
iced cheese	1	42	395
raspberry	1	62	414
Egg McMuffin	1	31	340
English muffin w/butter	1	30	186
hash brown potatoes	1 serving	15	144
hotcakes w/butter syrup	1 serving	94	500
pork sausage	1 serving	1	210
Sausage McMuffin	1	30	427
w/egg	1	32	517
scrambled eggs	1 serving	3	180
BURGERS & SANDWICHES			
Big Mac	1	39	570
cheeseburger	1	29	318
Filet-o-Fish	1	36	435
hamburger	1	28	263
McD.L.T.	1	40	680
Quarter Pounder	1	29	427
w/cheese	1	31	525
CHICKEN NUGGETS & SAUCES			
Chicken McNuggets	2	15	323
barbecue sauce	1 serving	14	60
honey	1 serving	12	50
hot mustard sauce	1 serving	11	63
sweet & sour sauce	1 serving	15	64
DESSERTS			
apple pie	1 piece	29	253
cookies			
Chocolaty Chip	1 serving	45	342
McDonaldland	1 serving	49	308
soft-serve ice cream & cone	1 serving	31	189
sundaes			
hot caramel	1	61	361
hot fudge	1	58	357
strawberry	1	54	320
SALAD BAR ITEMS			
bacon bits	1 serving	tr	15
chef salad	1	6	226
chicken salad Oriental	1	5	146
chow mein noodles	1 serving	5	45
croutons	1 serving	7	52
garden salad	1	4	91
shrimp salad	1	5	99
side salad	1	3	48

	Portion	Carbohydrates (g)	Total Calories
SALAD DRESSINGS			
bleu cheese	½ pkg	3	171
French	½ pkg	5	114
house	½ pkg	2	163
lite vinaigrette	½ pkg	3	25
Oriental	½ pkg	12	51
Thousand Island	½ pkg	5	198
SHAKES			
chocolate	1	66	383
strawberry	1	62	362
vanilla	1	60	352
SIDE DISHES			
french fries	1 regular serving	26	220
Roy Rogers			
BEVERAGES			
hot chocolate	1	22	123
BREAKFAST ITEMS			
crescent roll	1	27	287
crescent sandwich	1	25	401
w/bacon	1	26	431
w/ham	1	25	557
w/sausage	1	26	449
egg & biscuit platter	1	22	394
w/bacon	1	22	435
w/ham	1	23	442
w/sausage	1	22	550
pancake platter, w/syrup & butter	1	72	452
w/bacon	1	72	493
w/ham	1	72	506
w/sausage	1	72	608
BURGERS & SANDWICHES			
bacon cheeseburger	1	25	581
cheeseburger	1	27	563
hamburger	1	27	456
roast beef			
regular	1	29	317
w/cheese	1	30	424
large	1	30	360
w/cheese	1	30	467
RR Bar Burger	1	28	611

	Portion	Carbohydrates (g)	Total Calories
CHICKEN			
breast	1	17	412
breast & wing	1 each	25	604
drumstick/leg	1	6	140
nuggets	6	?	267
thigh	1	12	296
thigh & leg	1 each	17	436
wing	1	9	192
DESSERTS			
brownie	1	37	264
danish			
apple	1	32	249
cheese	1	31	254
cherry	1	32	271
strawberry shortcake	1 serving	59	447
sundaes			
caramel	1	52	293
hot fudge	1	53	337
strawberry	1	33	216
SALAD BAR ITEMS			
bacon bits	1 T	2	33
beets, sliced	¼ c	4	16
broccoli	½ c	4	20
carrots, shredded	¼ c	10	42
cheddar cheese	¼ c	1	112
Chinese noodles	¼ c	7	55
croutons	2 T	14	70
cucumbers	5–6 slices	1	4
eggs, chopped	2 T	1	55
green peas	¼ c	1	7
green peppers	¼ c	1	4
lettuce	1 c	4	10
macaroni salad	2 T	6	60
mushrooms	¼ c	1	5
potato salad	2 T	6	50
sunflower seeds	2 T	?	157
tomatoes	3 slices	5	20
SALAD DRESSINGS			
bacon & tomato	2 T	6	136
bleu cheese	2 T	2	150
low-cal Italian	2 T	2	70
Ranch	2 T	4	155
Thousand Island	2 T	4	160

	Portion	Carbohydrates (g)	Total Calories
SHAKES			
chocolate	1	61	358
strawberry	1	49	315
vanilla	1	45	306
SIDE DISHES			
biscuit	1	26	231
cole slaw	1 serving	11	110
french fries	1 regular serving	32	268
	1 large serving	43	357
hot topped potato			
plain	1	48	211
w/bacon & cheese	1	33	397
w/broccoli & cheese	1	40	376
w/oleo	1	48	274
w/sour cream & chives	1	48	408
w/taco beef & cheese	1	45	463
macaroni	1 serving	19	186
potato salad	1 serving	11	107
Wendy's			
BEVERAGES			
hot chocolate	1	23	110
lemonade	1	40	160
BREAKFAST ITEMS			
bacon	1 strip	<1	30
breakfast sandwich	1	33	370
buttermilk biscuit	1	37	320
danish			
apple	1	53	360
cheese	1	52	430
cinnamon raisin	1	55	410
French toast	2 slices	45	400
French toast toppings			
apple	1 pkt	32	130
blueberry	1 pkt	15	60
fried egg	1	1	90
grape jelly	1 pkt	10	40
omelet #1: ham & cheese	1	7	290
omelet #2: ham, cheese, & mushroom	1	0	250
omelet #3: ham, cheese, onion, & green pepper	1	7	280
omelet #4: mushroom, green pepper, & onion	1	7	210
potatoes	1 serving	37	360
sausage gravy	6 oz	13	440
sausage patty	1	<1	200

	Portion	Carbohydrates (g)	Total Calories
scrambled eggs	2 eggs	7	190
strawberry jam	1 pkt	10	40
syrup	1 pkt	37	140
toast, w/margarine			
wheat	2 slices	23	190
white	2 slices	35	250

BURGER & SANDWICH COMPONENTS

American cheese slice	1	<1	60
bacon	1 strip	<1	30
buns			
kaiser	1	32	180
multigrain	1	23	140
white	1	26	140
catsup	1 t	1	6
hamburger patty, ¼ lb	1	<1	210
lettuce	1 leaf	<1	2
mayonnaise	1 T	<1	90
mustard	1 t	<1	4
onion	3 rings	<1	2
pickles, dill	4 slices	<1	2
taco sauce	1 pkt	<1	10
tartar sauce	1 T	<1	80
tomatoes	1 slice	<1	2

BURGERS & SANDWICHES

Big Classic (two ¼-lb hamburger patties, mayonnaise, catsup, pickles, onion, tomatoes, lettuce, kaiser bun)	1	36	470
chicken breast fillet	1	4	200
chicken fried steak	1	25	580
fish fillet	1	13	210
Kids' Meal Hamburger	1	17	200

CHICKEN NUGGETS & SAUCES

Crispy Nuggets			
cooked in animal/vegetable oil	6	11	290
cooked in vegetable oil	6	14	310
barbecue sauce	1 pkt	11	50
honey	1 pkt	12	45
sweet & sour sauce	1 pkt	11	45
sweet mustard sauce	1 pkt	9	50

CHILI

chili	1 regular serving	24	240

	Portion	Carbohydrates (g)	Total Calories
CONDIMENTS, SAUCES, & MISCELLANEOUS ITEMS			
catsup	1 pkt	3	12
cheese sauce	2 oz	3	140
half & half	⅜ oz	<1	14
hot chili seasoning	1 pkt	2	6
margarine			
liquid	½ oz	<1	100
whipped	1 T	<1	70
nondairy creamer	⅜ oz	1	14
saltines	2	4	25
sour cream	2 t	<1	20
sugar	1 pkt	4	14
DESSERTS			
chocolate chip cookie	1	40	320
Frosty dairy dessert	1 regular serving	59	400
SALAD BAR ITEMS			
alfalfa sprouts	1 oz	<1	8
American cheese	1 oz	<1	90
bacon bits	⅛ oz	<1	10
blueberries	1 T	1	6
bread sticks	2	6	35
broccoli	½ c	2	12
cabbage, red	¼ c	<1	4
cantaloupe	2 pieces	4	18
carrots	¼ c	2	10
cauliflower	½ c	2	12
celery	1 T	<1	0
cheddar cheese	1 oz	<1	80
cherry peppers	1 T	<1	6
chow mein noodles	½ oz	8	70
cole slaw	¼ c	9	80
cottage cheese	½ c	3	110
croutons	½ oz	8	60
cucumbers	4 slices	<1	2
eggs	1 T	<1	30
grapefruit	2 oz	2	10
grapes	¼ c	7	30
green peas	1 oz	4	25
green peppers	¼ c	1	8
honeydew melon	2 pieces	5	20
jalapeño peppers	1 T	2	9
lettuce			
iceberg	1 c	1	8
romaine	1 c	1	10
mozzarella cheese	1 oz	<1	90
mushrooms	¼ c	<1	4
oranges	2 oz	7	25

	Portion	Carbohydrates (g)	Total Calories
Parmesan cheese, grated	1 oz	1	130
pasta salad	¼ c	18	130
peaches	2 slices	4	17
pepper rings	1 T	<1	2
pineapple chunks	½ c	18	70
provolone cheese	1 oz	<1	90
radishes	½ oz	<1	2
red onions	3 rings	<1	2
strawberries	2 oz	4	18
sunflower seeds & raisins	1 oz	6	140
Swiss cheese	1 oz	<1	90
tomatoes	1 oz	1	6
turkey ham	¼ c	<1	50
watermelon	2 pieces	4	18

SALAD DRESSINGS

Regular

bleu cheese	1 T	<1	60
celery seed	1 T	3	70
French style	1 T	5	70
Golden Italian	1 T	3	50
oil	1 T	<1	120
Ranch	1 T	<1	50
Thousand Island	1 T	2	70
wine vinegar	1 T	<1	2

Reduced-Calorie

bacon/tomato	1 T	2	45
creamy cucumber	1 T	2	50
Italian	1 T	2	25
Thousand Island	1 T	2	45

SIDE DISHES

french fries			
cooked in animal/vegetable oil	1 regular serving	38	310
cooked in vegetable oil	1 regular serving	35	300
hot stuffed baked potatoes			
plain	1	52	250
bacon & cheese	1	57	570
broccoli & cheese	1	54	500
cheese	1	55	590
chili & cheese	1	63	510
sour cream & chives	1	53	460

TACO SALAD

taco salad	1 serving	43	430
taco sauce	1 pkt	<1	10

	Portion	Carbohydrates (g)	Total Calories

❏ FATS, OILS, & SHORTENINGS
See also BUTTER & MARGARINE SPREADS

animal fats, all	1 T	0	115–116
shortening			
special for confectionery: frac-	1 T	0	120
tionated palm	1 c	0	1,927
all other	1 T	0	113–115
	1 c	0	1,812–1,845
vegetable oils, all	1 T	0	120

▪ BRAND NAME

Arrowhead Mills
all oils	1 T	0	120
Mazola			
corn oil	1 T	0	120
No-Stick	2½-second spray	0	6
Planters			
peanut oil	1 T	0	120
Rokeach			
Neutral Nyafat	1 T	0	99

❏ FISH *See* SEAFOOD & SEAFOOD PRODUCTS

❏ FLOURS & CORNMEALS
See also NUTS & NUT-BASED BUTTERS, FLOURS, MEALS, MILKS, PASTES, & POWDERS; SEEDS & SEED-BASED BUTTERS, FLOURS, & MEALS

arrowroot flour	1 T	7	29
barley flour	1 T	6	28
	1 c	86	401
buckwheat flour			
dark	1 oz	20	92
light, sifted	1 c	78	340
carob flour	1 T	7	14
	1 c	92	185

	Portion	Carbohydrates (g)	Total Calories
corn flour, sifted	1 c	85	405
masa harina	⅓ c	27	137
masa trigo	⅓ c	25	149
white, tortilla, lime-treated	1 oz	21	103
yellow, tortilla, untreated	1 oz	21	101
corn germ, toasted	1 oz	12	130
cornmeal			
whole-ground, dry			
bolted	1 c	91	122
unbolted	1 c	90	122
degermed, enriched			
dry	1 c	108	138
cooked	1 c	26	240
white, self-rising, dry	1 oz or ⅙ c	21	98
cornstarch	1 T	8	35
manioc (casava) flour	3½ oz	81	320
potato flour	1 c	143	628
rice bran	1 oz	16	80
rice flour	1 c	107	479
rice polish	1 oz	17	101
rye flour			
dark	3½ oz	68	327
light	3½ oz	78	357
rye wheat flour	1 c	86	400
soy flour *See* SOYBEANS & SOYBEAN PRODUCTS			
wheat & gluten flour	1 c	66	529
wheat flour, enriched			
all purpose			
sifted	1 c	88	420
unsifted	1 c	95	455
bread, sifted	1 c	84	409
cake or pastry, sifted	1 c	76	350
self-rising, unsifted	1 c	93	440
whole-wheat & soy flour	3½ oz	57	365
whole-wheat flour, from hard wheats	1 c	85	400
whole-wheat flour, straight, soft	3½ oz	77	364

• BRAND NAME

Argo
Argo & Kingsford's corn starch	1 T	7	30

Arrowhead Mills
barley flour	2 oz	43	200
brown rice flour	2 oz	44	200
buckwheat flour	2 oz	41	190
corn flour, yellow	2 oz	43	210

	Portion	Carbohydrates (g)	Total Calories
cornmeal			
blue	2 oz	41	210
hi-lysine	2 oz	43	210
yellow	2 oz	43	210
Ezekiel flour	2 oz	40	200
garbanzo flour	2 oz	35	200
millet flour	2 oz	41	185
oat flour	2 oz	43	200
pastry flour	2 oz	41	180
rye flour	2 oz	39	190
triticale flour	2 oz	41	190
unbleached white flour	2 oz	53	200
vital wheat gluten	1 oz	9	100
whole-wheat flour	2 oz	40	200
Aunt Jemima			
CORNMEAL			
bolted white, mix	⅙ c	21	99
bolted yellow, mix	⅙ c	21	97
buttermilk self-rising white, mix	3 T	20	101
enriched white	3 T	22	102
enriched yellow	3 T	22	102
self-rising white	⅙ c	21	98
self-rising white enriched bolted	⅙ c	20	99
FLOUR			
enriched self-rising	¼ c	24	109
Fearn			
rice flour	½ c	60	270
Featherweight			
potato starch	1 c	154	620
rice flour	1 c	113	500
Heckers			
flour	about 1 c or 4 oz	80–85	380–400
Quaker Oats			
masa harina de maiz	⅓ c	27	137
masa trigo	⅓ c	25	149

□ **FRANKFURTERS** *See* **PROCESSED MEAT & POULTRY PRODUCTS**

	Portion	Carbohydrates (g)	Total Calories

❑ FRUIT, FRESH & PROCESSED
See also PICKLES, OLIVES, RELISHES, & CHUTNEYS; SNACKS

	Portion	Carbohydrates (g)	Total Calories
acerolas, raw	1 c	8	31
apples			
raw			
w/skin	1 fruit = 4.9 oz	21	81
w/out skin	1 fruit = 4½ oz	19	72
baked in microwave, w/out skin	½ c sliced	12	48
boiled, w/out skin	½ c sliced	12	46
canned, sweetened, unheated	½ c sliced	17	68
dehydrated, sulfured			
cooked	½ c	19	71
uncooked	½ c	28	104
dried, sulfured			
cooked, w/added sugar	½ c	29	116
cooked, w/out added sugar	½ c	20	72
uncooked	2¼ oz	42	155
	1 c	57	209
frozen, unsweetened			
heated	½ c sliced	12	48
unheated	½ c sliced	11	41
applesauce, canned			
sweetened	½ c	25	97
unsweetened	½ c	14	53
apricots			
raw	3 fruit = 3.7 oz	12	51
canned, w/skin			
in water	3 halves + 1¾ T liquid	5	22
in juice	3 halves + 1¾ T liquid	10	40
in extra light syrup	3 halves + 1¾ T liquid	11	41
in light syrup	3 halves + 1¾ T liquid	14	54
in heavy syrup	3 halves + 1¾ T liquid	18	70
canned, w/out skin			
in water	2 fruit + 2 T liquid	5	20
in heavy syrup	2 fruit + 2 T liquid	19	75
in extra heavy syrup	2 fruit + 2 T liquid	22	87

	Portion	Carbohydrates (g)	Total Calories
dehydrated (low-moisture), sulfured			
cooked	½ c	40	156
uncooked	½ c	50	192
dried, sulfured			
cooked, w/added sugar	½ c halves	39	153
cooked, w/out added sugar	½ c halves	27	106
uncooked	10 halves	22	83
frozen, sweetened	½ c	30	119
avocados, raw			
all commercial varieties	1 fruit = 7.1 oz	15	324
	1 c puree	17	370
California	1 fruit = 6.1 oz	12	306
	1 c puree	16	407
Florida	1 fruit = 10.7 oz	27	339
	1 c puree	21	257
bananas			
raw	1 fruit = 4 oz	27	105
dehydrated (banana powder)	1 T	5	21
blackberries			
raw	½ c	9	37
canned, in heavy syrup	½ c	30	118
frozen, unsweetened	1 c	24	97
blueberries			
raw	1 c	20	82
canned, in heavy syrup	½ c	28	112
frozen			
sweetened	1 c	50	187
unsweetened	1 c	19	78
boysenberries			
canned, in heavy syrup	½ c	29	113
frozen, unsweetened	1 c	16	66
breadfruit, raw	¼ small fruit = 3.4 oz	26	99
candied fruit See BAKING INGREDIENTS			
cantaloupe See melons, below			
carambolas, raw	1 fruit = 4½ oz	10	42
carissa plums, raw	1 fruit = 0.7 oz	3	12
casaba See melons, below			
cherimoyas, raw	1 fruit = 19¼ oz	131	515
cherries, sour, red			
raw	1 c w/pits	13	51
canned			
in water	½ c	11	43
in light syrup	½ c	24	94

	Portion	Carbohydrates (g)	Total Calories
cherries, sour, red: canned *(cont.)*			
in heavy syrup	½ c	30	116
in extra heavy syrup	½ c	38	148
frozen, unsweetened	1 c	17	72
cherries, sweet			
raw	10 fruit = 2.4 oz	11	49
canned			
in water	½ c	15	57
in juice	½ c	17	68
in light syrup	½ c	22	85
in heavy syrup	½ c	27	107
in extra heavy syrup	½ c	34	133
frozen, sweetened	1 c	58	232
Chinese gooseberries *See* kiwi fruit, *below*			
coconut *See* BAKING INGREDIENTS; NUTS & NUT-BASED BUTTERS, FLOURS, MEALS, MILKS, PASTES, & POWDERS			
crabapples, raw	1 c sliced	22	83
cranberries, raw	1 c whole	12	46
cranberry sauce, canned, sweetened	½ c	54	209
currants			
European, black, raw	½ c	9	36
red & white, raw	½ c	8	31
zante, dried	½ c	53	204
custard apples, raw	edible portion = 3½ oz	25	101
dates, domestic, dry	10 fruit = 2.9 oz	61	228
elderberries, raw	1 c	27	105
figs			
raw	1 medium fruit = 1¾ oz	10	37
canned			
in water	3 fruit + 1¾ T liquid	11	42
in light syrup	3 fruit + 1¾ T liquid	15	58
in heavy syrup	3 fruit + 1¾ T liquid	19	75
in extra heavy syrup	3 fruit + 1¾ T liquid	29	91
dried			
cooked	½ c	36	140
uncooked	10 fruit = 6.6 oz	122	477
fruit cocktail, canned			
in water	½ c	10	40
in juice	½ c	15	56
in extra light syrup	½ c	14	55
in light syrup	½ c	19	72

	Portion	Carbohydrates (g)	Total Calories
in heavy syrup	½ c	24	93
in extra heavy syrup	½ c	30	115
fruit salad, canned			
in water	½ c	10	37
in juice	½ c	16	62
in light syrup	½ c	19	73
in heavy syrup	½ c	24	94
in extra heavy syrup	½ c	30	114
fruit salad, tropical, canned, in heavy syrup	½ c	29	110
gooseberries			
raw	1 c	15	67
canned, in light syrup	½ c	24	93
grandillas See passion fruit, below			
grapefruit			
raw, pink & red	½ fruit = 4.3 oz	10	37
raw, white	½ fruit = 4.2 oz	10	39
canned			
in water	½ c	11	44
in juice	½ c	11	46
in light syrup	½ c	20	76
grapes			
American type, raw	10 fruit = 0.8 oz	4	15
European type, raw	10 fruit = 1.8 oz	9	36
Thompson seedless, canned			
in water	½ c	13	48
in heavy syrup, solids & liquids	½ c	25	94
groundcherries, raw	½ c	8	37
guavas			
common, raw	1 fruit = 3.2 oz	11	45
strawberry, raw	1 fruit = 0.2 oz	1	4
guava sauce, cooked	½ c	11	43
honeydew See melons, below			
jackfruit, raw	edible portion = 3½ oz	24	94
jujubes			
raw	edible portion = 3½ oz	20	79
dried	edible portion = 3½ oz	74	287
kiwi fruit, raw	1 medium fruit = 2.7 oz	11	46
kumquats, raw	1 fruit = 0.7 oz	3	12

	Portion	Carbohydrates (g)	Total Calories
lemon peel, raw	1 t	tr	?
	1 T	1	?
lemons, raw			
w/peel	1 medium fruit = 3.8 oz	12	22
w/out peel	1 medium fruit = 2 oz	5	17
limes, raw	1 fruit = 2.4 oz	7	20
litchis *See* lychees, *below*			
loganberries, frozen	1 c	19	80
longans			
raw	1 fruit = 0.1 oz	tr	2
dried	edible portion = 3½ oz	74	286
loquats, raw	1 fruit = 0.3 oz	1	5
lychees			
raw	1 fruit = 0.3 oz	2	6
dried	edible portion = 3½ oz	71	277
mammy apples, raw	1 fruit = 29.8 oz	106	431
mangos, raw	1 fruit = 7.3 oz	35	135
melon balls, frozen, cantaloupe & honeydew	1 c	14	55
melons			
cantaloupe, raw	½ fruit = 9.4 oz	22	94
	1 c cubed	13	57
casaba, raw	1/10 fruit = 5.8 oz	10	43
	1 c cubed	11	45
honeydew, raw	1/10 fruit = 4½ oz	12	46
	1 c cubed	16	60
muskmelon *See* cantaloupe, *above*			
mixed fruit			
canned, in heavy syrup, solids & liquids	½ c	24	92
dried	11 oz	188	712
frozen, sweetened	1 c	61	245
mulberries, raw	10 fruit = ½ oz	1	7
muskmelons *See* melons: cantaloupe, *above*			
natal plums *See* carissa plums, *above*			

	Portion	Carbohydrates (g)	Total Calories
nectarines, raw	1 fruit = 4.8 oz	16	67
oheloberries, raw	10 fruit = 0.4 oz	1	3
orange peel, raw	1 t	1	?
	1 T	2	?
oranges, raw			
w/peel	1 fruit = 5.6 oz	25	64
w/out peel			
all commercial varieties	1 fruit = 4.6 oz	15	62
California, navels	1 fruit = 4.9 oz	16	65
California, Valencias	1 fruit = 4.3 oz	14	59
Florida	1 fruit = 5.3 oz	17	69
papayas, raw	1 fruit = 10.7 oz	30	117
passion fruit, purple, raw	1 fruit = 0.6 oz	4	18
peaches			
raw	1 fruit = 3.1 oz	10	37
canned, clingstone			
in water	1 half + 1⅔ T liquid	5	18
in extra light syrup	1 half + 1⅔ T liquid	9	32
in light syrup	1 half + 1¾ T liquid	12	44
canned, clingstone & freestone			
in juice	1 half + 1⅔ T liquid	9	34
in heavy syrup	1 half + 1¾ T liquid	16	60
canned, freestone, in extra heavy syrup	1 half + 1¾ T liquid	21	77
dehydrated (low-moisture), sulfured			
cooked	½ c	41	161
uncooked	½ c	48	188
dried, sulfured			
cooked, w/added sugar	½ c halves	36	139
cooked, w/out added sugar	½ c halves	25	99
uncooked	10 halves	80	311
frozen, sweetened	1 c sliced, thawed	60	235

	Portion	Carbohydrates (g)	Total Calories
peaches, spiced, canned, in heavy syrup	1 fruit + 2 T liquid	18	66
pears			
raw	1 fruit = 5.8 oz	25	98
canned			
in water	1 half + 1⅔ T liquid	6	22
in juice	1 half + 1⅔ T liquid	10	38
in extra light syrup	1 half + 1⅔ T liquid	9	36
in light syrup	1 half + 1¾ T liquid	12	45
in heavy syrup	1 half + 1¾ T liquid	15	58
in extra heavy syrup	1 half + 1¾ T liquid	20	77
dried, sulfured			
cooked, w/added sugar	½ c halves	52	196
cooked, w/out added sugar	½ c halves	43	163
uncooked	10 halves	122	459
persimmons			
Japanese			
raw	1 fruit = 5.9 oz	31	118
dried	1 fruit = 1.2 oz	25	93
native, raw	1 fruit = 0.9 oz	8	32
pineapple			
raw	1 slice = 3 oz	10	42
	1 c diced	19	77
canned			
in water	1 slice + 1¼ T liquid	5	19
	1 c tidbits	20	79
in juice	1 slice + 1¼ T liquid	9	35
	1 c chunks or tidbits	39	150
in light syrup	1 slice + 1¼ T liquid	8	30
	1 c	34	131
in heavy syrup	1 slice + 1¼ T liquid	12	45
	1 c chunks, tidbits, or crushed	52	199

	Portion	Carbohydrates (g)	Total Calories
in extra heavy syrup	1 slice + 1¼ T liquid	12	48
	1 c chunks or crushed	56	217
frozen, sweetened	½ c chunks	27	104
pitangas, raw	1 fruit = 0.2 oz	1	2
	1 c	13	57
plantains			
raw	1 fruit = 6.3 oz	57	218
cooked	½ c sliced	24	89
plums, purple			
raw	1 fruit = 2.3 oz	9	36
canned			
in water	3 fruit + 2 T liquid	10	39
	1 c	27	102
in juice	3 fruit + 2 T liquid	14	55
	1 c	38	146
in light syrup	3 fruit + 2¾ T liquid	22	83
	1 c	41	158
in heavy syrup	3 fruit + 2¾ T liquid	31	119
	1 c	61	230
in extra heavy syrup	3 fruit + 2¾ T liquid	35	135
	1 c	69	265
pomegranates, raw	1 fruit = 5.4 oz	26	104
prickly pears, raw	1 fruit = 3.6 oz	10	42
prunes			
canned, in heavy syrup	5 fruit + 2 T liquid	24	90
	1 c	65	245
dehydrated (low-moisture)			
cooked	½ c	42	158
uncooked	½ c	59	224
dried			
cooked, w/added sugar	½ c	39	147
cooked, w/out added sugar	½ c	30	113
uncooked	10 fruit = 3 oz	53	201
	1 c	101	385
pummelos, raw	1 fruit = 21.4 oz	59	228
	1 c sections	18	71

	Portion	Carbohydrates (g)	Total Calories
quinces, raw	1 fruit = 3.2 oz	14	53
raisins			
golden seedless	1 c not packed	115	437
	1 c packed	131	498
seeded	1 c not packed	114	428
	1 c packed	129	488
seedless	1 c not packed	115	434
	1 c packed	131	494
raspberries, red			
raw	1 c	14	61
canned, in heavy syrup, solids & liquids	½ c	30	117
frozen, sweetened	1 c	tr	256
	10 oz pkg	tr	291
rhubarb			
raw	½ c diced	3	13
frozen			
cooked, w/added sugar	½ c	37	139
uncooked	½ c	3	14
rose apples, raw	edible portion = 3½ oz	6	25
roselles, raw	1 c	6	28
sapodillas, raw	1 fruit = 6 oz	34	140
sapotes, raw	1 fruit = 7.9 oz	76	301
soursops, raw	1 fruit = 22 oz	105	416
starfruit See carambolas, above			
strawberries			
raw	1 c	10	45
canned, in heavy syrup	½ c	30	117
frozen, sweetened			
sliced	1 c	66	245
	10 oz pkg	74	273
whole	1 c	54	200
	10 oz pkg	60	223
frozen, unsweetened	1 c	14	52
sugar apples, raw	1 fruit = 5½ oz	37	146
Surinam cherries See pitangas, above			
sweetsop See sugar apples, above			
tamarinds, raw	1 fruit = 0.1 oz	1	5
tangerines			
raw	1 fruit = 3 oz	9	37

	Portion	Carbohydrates (g)	Total Calories
canned			
in juice, solids & liquids	½ c	12	46
in light syrup, solids & liquids	½ c	20	76
watermelon, raw	¹⁄₁₆ fruit = 17 oz	35	152
	1 c diced	11	50

West Indian cherries *See* acerolas, *above*

- ## BRAND NAME

Birds Eye

mixed fruit in syrup	5 oz	31	120
red raspberries in lite syrup	5 oz	25	100
strawberries, halved, in lite syrup	5 oz	22	90
strawberries, halved, in syrup	5 oz	30	120

Dole

mandarin oranges in light syrup	½ c	20	76
pineapple cuts in juice	½ c	18	70
pineapple cuts in syrup	½ c	25	95

Dromedary

chopped dates	¼ c	31	130
pitted dates	5	23	100

Fresh Chef

Tropical Delight fruit salad	7 oz	32	240

Mott's

applesauce	4 oz	22	88
chunky applesauce	4 oz	14	57
cinnamon applesauce	4 oz	18	72
natural applesauce	4 oz	11	44

Mrs. Paul's

apple fritters	2	36	270

Oregon Freeze Dry

banana chips	¼ c	14	124
fruit nuggets	½ c	?	?
peaches	½ c	12	45
strawberries	½ c	20	60

Stouffer

escalloped apples	4 oz	28	140

❑ FRUIT & NUT SNACK MIXES
See SNACKS

	Portion	Carbohydrates (g)	Total Calories

❏ FRUIT CHUTNEYS & RELISHES *See* PICKLES, OLIVES, RELISHES, & CHUTNEYS

❏ FRUIT SAUCES *See* FRUIT, FRESH & PROCESSED

❏ FRUIT SPREADS

Fruit Butters

	Portion	Carbohydrates (g)	Total Calories
apple	1 T	9	37
guava	1 T	10	39

Jams

	Portion	Carbohydrates (g)	Total Calories
average, all varieties			
regular	1 T	14	55
low-cal	1 T	7	29
grape	1 T	15	59
plum	1 T	15	59

Jellies

	Portion	Carbohydrates (g)	Total Calories
average, all varieties			
regular	1 T	14	55
low-cal	1 T	7	27
blackberry	1 T	13	51
boysenberry	1 T	13	52
cherry	1 T	13	52
currant	1 T	13	52
grape	1 T	14	55
guava	1 T	13	52
quince	1 T	13	51
strawberry	1 T	13	51

Marmalades

	Portion	Carbohydrates (g)	Total Calories
citrus	1 T	14	51
orange	1 T	14	56
papaya	1 T	15	57

Preserves

	Portion	Carbohydrates (g)	Total Calories
apricot	1 T	13	51
apricot-pineapple	1 T	13	51
blackberry	1 T	14	55
boysenberry	1 T	14	54
peach	1 T	13	51

	Portion	Carbohydrates (g)	Total Calories

● **BRAND NAME**

Smucker's
FRUIT BUTTERS

apple	2 t	6	25
peach	2 t	8	30

JAMS, JELLIES, MARMALADES, & PRESERVES

all jams, jellies, & preserves			
regular	2 t	9	35
low-sugar or Slenderella	2 t	4	16
imitation grape jelly or straw-berry jam, artificially swee-tened	2 t	1	4
orange marmalade	2 t	9	35

❑ **GELATIN & GELATIN DESSERTS** *See* DESSERTS: CUSTARDS, GELATINS, PUDDINGS, & PIE FILLINGS

❑ **GRAINS** *See* RICE & GRAINS, PLAIN & PREPARED

❑ **GRAVIES** *See* SAUCES, GRAVIES, & CONDIMENTS

❑ **HAM** *See* PORK, FRESH & CURED; PROCESSED MEAT & POULTRY PRODUCTS

❑ **HERBS & SPICES** *See* SEASONINGS

❑ **HONEY** *See* SUGARS & SWEETENERS

❑ **HOT DOGS** *See* frankfurters, *under* PROCESSED MEAT & POULTRY PRODUCTS

❑ **ICE CREAM & ICE MILK** *See* DESSERTS, FROZEN

	Portion	Carbohydrates (g)	Total Calories

INFANT & TODDLER FOODS

Baked Products

arrowroot cookies	1	4	24
	1 oz	20	125
pretzels	1	5	24
	1 oz	23	113
teething biscuits	1	8	43
	1 oz	22	111
zwieback	1	5	30
	1 oz	21	121

Cereals, Hot & Cold

barley			
dry	½ oz	11	52
	1 T	2	9
w/whole milk	1 oz	5	31
cereal & egg yolks			
strained	about 4½ oz	9	66
	1 oz	2	15
junior	about 7½ oz	15	110
	1 oz	2	15
cereal, egg yolks, & bacon			
strained	about 4½ oz	8	101
	1 oz	2	22
junior	about 7½ oz	15	178
	1 oz	2	24
high protein			
dry	½ oz	7	51
	1 T	1	9
w/whole milk	1 oz	3	31
high protein w/apple & orange			
dry	½ oz	8	53
	1 T	1	9
w/whole milk	1 oz	4	32
mixed			
dry	½ oz	10	54
	1 T	2	9
w/whole milk	1 oz	5	32
mixed w/applesauce & ba-nanas			
strained	about 4.8 oz	24	111
	1 oz	5	23
junior	about 7.8 oz	41	183
	1 oz	5	24
mixed w/bananas			
dry	½ oz	11	56
	1 T	2	9

	Portion	Carbohydrates (g)	Total Calories
w/whole milk	1 oz	5	33
mixed w/honey			
dry	½ oz	10	55
	1 T	2	9
w/whole milk	1 oz	5	33
oatmeal			
dry	½ oz	10	56
	1 T	2	10
w/whole milk	1 oz	4	33
oatmeal w/applesauce & bananas			
strained	about 4.8 oz	21	99
	1 oz	4	21
junior	about 7.8 oz	35	165
	1 oz	5	21
oatmeal w/bananas			
dry	½ oz	10	56
	1 T	2	9
w/whole milk	1 oz	5	33
oatmeal w/honey			
dry	½ oz	10	55
	1 T	2	9
w/whole milk	1 oz	4	33
rice			
dry	½ oz	11	56
	1 T	2	9
w/whole milk	1 oz	5	33
rice w/applesauce & bananas, strained	about 4.8 oz	23	107
	1 oz	5	23
rice w/bananas			
dry	½ oz	11	57
	1 T	2	10
w/whole milk	1 oz	5	33
rice w/honey			
dry	½ oz	11	56
	1 T	2	9
w/whole milk	1 oz	5	33
rice w/mixed fruit, junior	about 7.8 oz	41	186
	1 oz	5	24

Desserts

apple Betty			
strained	about 4.8 oz	27	97
	1 oz	6	20
junior	about 7.8 oz	42	153
	1 oz	5	20
caramel pudding			
strained	about 4.8 oz	23	104
	1 oz	5	22

	Portion	Carbohydrates (g)	Total Calories
caramel pudding *(cont.)*			
junior	about 7½ oz	36	167
	1 oz	5	22
cherry vanilla pudding			
strained	about 4.8 oz	24	91
	1 oz	5	19
junior	about 7.8 oz	41	152
	1 oz	5	20
chocolate custard pudding			
strained	about 4½ oz	21	107
	1 oz	5	24
junior	about 7.8 oz	38	195
	1 oz	5	25
cottage cheese w/pineapple			
strained	about 4.8 oz	18	94
	1 oz	4	20
junior	about 7.8 oz	35	172
	1 oz	5	22
Dutch apple			
strained	about 4.8 oz	23	92
	1 oz	5	19
junior	about 7.8 oz	37	151
	1 oz	5	19
fruit dessert			
strained	about 4.8 oz	22	79
	1 oz	5	17
junior	about 7.8 oz	38	138
	1 oz	5	18
orange pudding, strained	about 4.8 oz	24	108
	1 oz	5	23
peach cobbler			
strained	about 4.8 oz	24	88
	1 oz	5	18
junior	about 7.8 oz	40	147
	1 oz	5	19
peach melba			
strained	about 4.8 oz	22	81
	1 oz	5	17
junior	about 7.8 oz	36	132
	1 oz	5	17
pineapple orange, strained	about 4½ oz	24	89
	1 oz	5	20
pineapple pudding			
strained	about 4½ oz	26	104
	1 oz	6	23
junior	about 7.8 oz	47	192
	1 oz	6	25
tropical fruit, junior	about 7.8 oz	36	131
	1 oz	5	17
vanilla custard pudding			
strained	about 4½ oz	21	109
	1 oz	5	24

	Portion	Carbohydrates (g)	Total Calories
junior	about 7.8 oz	36	196
	1 oz	5	25

Dinners, Regular

	Portion	Carbohydrates (g)	Total Calories
beef & egg noodles			
strained	about 4½ oz	9	68
	1 oz	2	15
junior	about 7½ oz	16	122
	1 oz	2	16
beef & rice, toddler	about 6.2 oz	16	146
	1 oz	3	23
beef lasagna, toddler	about 6.2 oz	18	137
	1 oz	3	22
beef stew, toddler	about 6.2 oz	10	90
	1 oz	2	14
chicken & noodles			
strained	about 4½ oz	10	67
	1 oz	2	15
junior	about 7½ oz	16	109
	1 oz	2	15
chicken soup, strained	about 4½ oz	9	64
	1 oz	2	14
chicken soup, cream of,	about 4½ oz	11	74
strained	1 oz	2	16
chicken stew, toddler	about 6 oz	11	132
	1 oz	2	22
lamb & noodles, junior	about 1½ oz	19	138
	1 oz	3	18
macaroni & bacon, toddler	about 7½ oz	18	160
	1 oz	2	21
macaroni & cheese			
strained	about 4½ oz	10	76
	1 oz	2	17
junior	about 7½ oz	18	130
	1 oz	2	17
macaroni & ham, junior	about 7½ oz	18	127
	1 oz	2	17
macaroni, tomato, & beef			
strained	about 4½ oz	11	71
	1 oz	3	16
junior	about 7½ oz	20	125
	1 oz	3	17
mixed vegetables			
strained	about 4½ oz	12	52
	1 oz	3	11
junior	about 7½ oz	17	71
	1 oz	2	9

	Portion	Carbohydrates (g)	Total Calories
spaghetti, tomato, & meat			
junior	about 7½ oz	22	135
	1 oz	3	18
toddler	about 6.2 oz	19	133
	1 oz	3	21
split peas & ham, junior	about 7½ oz	24	152
	1 oz	3	20
turkey & rice			
strained	about 4½ oz	9	63
	1 oz	2	14
junior	about 7½ oz	15	104
	1 oz	2	14
vegetables & bacon			
strained	about 4½ oz	11	88
	1 oz	2	19
junior	about 7½ oz	16	150
	1 oz	2	20
vegetables & beef			
strained	about 4½ oz	9	67
	1 oz	2	15
junior	about 7½ oz	16	113
	1 oz	2	15
vegetables & chicken			
strained	about 4½ oz	9	55
	1 oz	2	12
junior	about 7½ oz	18	106
	1 oz	2	14
vegetables & ham			
strained	about 4½ oz	9	62
	1 oz	2	14
junior	about 7½ oz	15	110
	1 oz	2	15
toddler	about 6.2 oz	14	128
	1 oz	2	21
vegetables & lamb			
strained	about 4½ oz	9	67
	1 oz	2	15
junior	about 7½ oz	15	108
	1 oz	2	14
vegetables & liver			
strained	about 4½ oz	9	50
	1 oz	2	11
junior	about 7½ oz	18	93
	1 oz	2	12
vegetables & turkey			
strained	about 4½ oz	8	54
	1 oz	2	12
junior	about 7½ oz	16	101
	1 oz	2	13

	Portion	Carbohydrates (g)	Total Calories
toddler	about 6.2 oz	14	141
	1 oz	2	23
vegetables, dumplings, & beef			
strained	about 4½ oz	10	61
	1 oz	2	14
junior	about 7½ oz	17	103
	1 oz	2	14
vegetables, noodles, & chicken			
strained	about 4½ oz	10	81
	1 oz	2	18
junior	about 7½ oz	19	137
	1 oz	3	18
vegetables, noodles, & turkey			
strained	about 4½ oz	9	56
	1 oz	2	12
junior	about 7½ oz	16	110
	1 oz	2	15

Dinners, High in Meat or Cheese

	Portion	Carbohydrates (g)	Total Calories
beef w/vegetables			
strained	about 4½ oz	5	96
	1 oz	1	21
junior	about 4½ oz	7	108
	1 oz	2	24
chicken w/vegetables			
strained	about 4½ oz	8	100
	1 oz	2	22
junior	about 4½ oz	5	117
	1 oz	1	26
cottage cheese w/pineapple,	about 4.8 oz	25	157
strained	1 oz	5	33
ham w/vegetables			
strained	about 4½ oz	7	97
	1 oz	2	21
junior	about 4½ oz	8	98
	1 oz	2	22
turkey w/vegetables			
strained	about 4½ oz	8	111
	1 oz	2	25
junior	about 4½ oz	8	115
	1 oz	2	25
veal w/vegetables			
strained	about 4½ oz	8	89
	1 oz	2	20
junior	about 4½ oz	7	93
	1 oz	2	21

	Portion	Carbohydrates (g)	Total Calories

Fruit
See also Desserts, *above*

	Portion	Carbohydrates (g)	Total Calories
apple blueberry			
strained	about 4.8 oz	22	82
	1 oz	5	17
junior	about 7.8 oz	37	137
	1 oz	5	18
apple raspberry			
strained	about 4.8 oz	21	79
	1 oz	5	17
junior	about 7.8 oz	34	127
	1 oz	4	16
applesauce			
strained	about 4½ oz	14	53
	1 oz	3	12
junior	about 7½ oz	22	79
	1 oz	3	11
applesauce & apricots			
strained	about 4.8 oz	16	60
	1 oz	3	13
junior	about 7.8 oz	27	104
	1 oz	4	13
applesauce & cherries			
strained	about 4.8 oz	18	65
	1 oz	4	14
junior	about 7.8 oz	29	106
	1 oz	4	14
applesauce & pineapple			
strained	about 4½ oz	13	48
	1 oz	3	11
junior	about 7½ oz	22	83
	1 oz	3	11
apricots w/tapioca			
strained	about 4.8 oz	22	80
	1 oz	5	17
junior	about 7.8 oz	38	139
	1 oz	5	18
bananas & pineapple w/tapioca			
strained	about 4.8 oz	25	91
	1 oz	5	19
junior	about 7.8 oz	39	143
	1 oz	5	18
bananas w/tapioca			
strained	about 4.8 oz	21	77
	1 oz	4	16
junior	about 7.8 oz	39	147
	1 oz	5	19
guava & papaya w/tapioca,	about 4½ oz	22	80
strained	1 oz	5	18

	Portion	Carbohydrates (g)	Total Calories
guava w/tapioca, strained	about 4½ oz	23	86
	1 oz	5	19
mango w/tapioca, strained	about 4.8 oz	29	109
	1 oz	6	23
papaya & applesauce w/tap- ioca, strained	about 4½ oz	24	89
	1 oz	5	20
peaches			
strained	about 4.8 oz	26	96
	1 oz	5	20
junior	about 7.8 oz	42	157
	1 oz	5	20
pears			
strained	about 4½ oz	14	53
	1 oz	3	12
junior	about 7½ oz	25	93
	1 oz	3	12
pears & pineapple			
strained	about 4½ oz	14	52
	1 oz	3	12
junior	about 7½ oz	24	93
	1 oz	3	12
plums w/tapioca			
strained	about 4.8 oz	27	96
	1 oz	6	20
junior	about 7.8 oz	45	163
	1 oz	6	21
prunes w/tapioca			
strained	about 4.8 oz	25	94
	1 oz	5	20
junior	about 7.8 oz	41	155
	1 oz	5	20

Fruit Juices

apple	about 4.2 oz	15	61
	1 fl oz	4	14
apple-cherry	about 4.2 oz	13	53
	1 fl oz	3	13
apple-grape	about 4.2 oz	15	60
	1 fl oz	4	14
apple-peach	about 4.2 oz	14	55
	1 fl oz	3	13
apple-plum	about 4.2 oz	16	63
	1 fl oz	4	15
apple-prune	about 4.2 oz	23	94
	1 fl oz	6	23
mixed fruit	about 4.2 oz	15	61
	1 fl oz	4	14
orange	about 4.2 oz	13	58
	1 fl oz	3	14

	Portion	Carbohydrates (g)	Total Calories
orange-apple	about 4.2 oz	13	56
	1 fl oz	3	13
orange-apple-banana	about 4.2 oz	15	61
	1 fl oz	4	15
orange-apricot	about 4.2 oz	14	60
	1 fl oz	3	14
orange-banana	about 4.2 oz	15	65
	1 fl oz	4	15
orange-pineapple	about 4.2 oz	15	63
	1 fl oz	4	15
prune-orange	about 4.2 oz	22	91
	1 fl oz	5	22

Meats & Egg Yolks

	Portion	Carbohydrates (g)	Total Calories
beef			
strained	about 3½ oz	0	106
	1 oz	0	30
junior	about 3½ oz	0	105
	1 oz	0	30
beef w/beef heart, strained	about 3½ oz	0	93
	1 oz	0	27
chicken			
strained	about 3½ oz	tr	128
	1 oz	0	37
junior	about 3½ oz	0	148
	1 oz	0	42
chicken sticks, junior	2½ oz	1	134
	1 stick = 0.35 oz	tr	19
egg yolks, strained	about 3.3 oz	1	191
	1 oz	tr	58
ham			
strained	about 3½ oz	0	110
	1 oz	0	32
junior	about 3½ oz	0	123
	1 oz	0	35
lamb			
strained	about 3½ oz	tr	102
	1 oz	0	29
junior	about 3½ oz	0	111
	1 oz	0	32
liver, strained	about 3½ oz	1	100
	1 oz	tr	29
meat sticks, junior	2½ oz	1	130
	1 stick = 0.35 oz	tr	18
pork, strained	about 3½ oz	0	123
	1 oz	0	35

	Portion	Carbohydrates (g)	Total Calories
turkey			
strained	about 3½ oz	tr	113
	1 oz	0	32
junior	about 3½ oz	0	128
	1 oz	0	37
turkey sticks, junior	2½ oz	1	129
	1 stick = 0.35 oz	tr	18
veal			
strained	about 3½ oz	0	100
	1 oz	0	29
junior	about 3½ oz	0	109
	1 oz	0	31

Vegetables

	Portion	Carbohydrates (g)	Total Calories
beans, green			
plain			
strained	about 4½ oz	8	32
	1 oz	2	7
junior	about 7.3 oz	12	51
	1 oz	2	7
buttered			
strained	about 4½ oz	9	42
	1 oz	2	9
junior	about 7.3 oz	13	67
	1 oz	2	9
creamed, junior	about 7½ oz	15	68
	1 oz	2	9
beets, strained	about 4½ oz	10	43
	1 oz	2	10
carrots			
plain			
strained	about 4½ oz	8	34
	1 oz	2	8
junior	about 7½ oz	15	67
	1 oz	2	9
buttered			
strained	about 4½ oz	9	46
	1 oz	2	10
junior	about 7½ oz	14	70
	1 oz	2	9
corn, creamed			
strained	about 4½ oz	18	73
	1 oz	4	16
junior	about 7½ oz	35	138
	1 oz	5	18
garden vegetables, strained	about 4½ oz	9	48
	1 oz	2	11

	Portion	Carbohydrates (g)	Total Calories
mixed vegetables			
strained	about 4½ oz	10	52
	1 oz	2	11
junior	about 7½ oz	17	88
	1 oz	2	12
peas			
plain, strained	about 4½ oz	10	52
	1 oz	2	11
buttered			
strained	about 4½ oz	14	72
	1 oz	3	16
junior	about 7.3 oz	23	123
	1 oz	3	17
creamed, strained	about 4½ oz	11	68
	1 oz	3	15
spinach, creamed			
strained	about 4½ oz	7	48
	1 oz	2	11
junior	about 7½ oz	14	90
	1 oz	2	12
squash			
plain			
strained	about 4½ oz	7	30
	1 oz	2	7
junior	about 7½ oz	12	51
	1 oz	2	7
buttered			
strained	about 4½ oz	9	37
	1 oz	2	8
junior	about 7½ oz	14	63
	1 oz	2	8
sweet potatoes			
plain			
strained	about 4.8 oz	18	77
	1 oz	4	16
junior	about 7.8 oz	31	133
	1 oz	4	17
buttered			
strained	about 4.8 oz	16	76
	1 oz	3	16
junior	about 7.8 oz	27	126
	1 oz	4	16

▪ BRAND NAME

Beech-Nut
STAGE 1

Cereal

barley	½ oz dry	10	50
	½ oz dry + 2.4 fl oz milk	14	100

	Portion	Carbohydrates (g)	Total Calories
oatmeal	½ oz dry	9	50
	½ oz dry + 2.4 fl oz milk	13	100
rice	½ oz dry	11	60
	½ oz dry + 2.4 fl oz milk	14	100
Fruit & Fruit Dishes			
bartlett pears	4½ oz	16	70
Chiquita bananas	4½ oz	24	100
golden delicious applesauce	4½ oz	14	60
yellow cling peaches	4½ oz	14	60
Fruit Juices			
apple	4.2 fl oz	14	60
pear	4.2 fl oz	14	60
white grape	4.2 fl oz	20	80
Meat			
beef	3½ oz	1	120
chicken	3½ oz	1	110
lamb	3½ oz	1	130
turkey	3⅓ oz	1	120
veal	3½ oz	1	120
Vegetables			
butternut squash	4½ oz	10	40
green beans	4½ oz	8	40
regal imperial carrots	4½ oz	9	40
sweet potatoes	4½ oz	16	70
tender sweet peas	4½ oz	12	70
STAGE 2			
Cereals			
Hi-Protein	½ oz dry	7	50
	½ oz dry + 2.4 fl oz milk	10	90
mixed	½ oz dry	10	50
	½ oz dry + 2.4 fl oz milk	13	100
w/applesauce & bananas	4½ oz	18	80
oatmeal			
w/applesauce & bananas	4½ oz	17	90
w/bananas	½ oz dry	11	60
	½ oz dry + 2.4 fl oz milk	14	100
rice			
w/applesauce & bananas	4½ oz	22	100

	Portion	Carbohydrates (g)	Total Calories
rice *(cont.)*			
w/bananas	½ oz dry	13	60
	½ oz dry + 2.4 fl oz milk	17	100
Desserts			
banana custard	4½ oz	26	120
banana pineapple	4½ oz	25	100
Dutch apple	4½ oz	20	80
guava tropical fruit	4½ oz	24	100
mango tropical fruit	4½ oz	23	90
papaya tropical fruit	4½ oz	20	80
vanilla custard	4½ oz	22	130
Fruit & Dairy			
cottage cheese w/pineapple	4½ oz	24	110
mixed fruit & yogurt	4½ oz	24	110
peaches & yogurt	4½ oz	25	110
Fruit & Fruit Dishes			
apples & grapes	4½ oz	22	90
apples & strawberries	4½ oz	22	90
applesauce & apricots	4½ oz	14	60
applesauce & bananas	4½ oz	15	60
applesauce & cherries	4½ oz	17	70
apples, mandarin oranges, & bananas	4½ oz	22	90
apples, peaches, & strawberries	4½ oz	24	100
apples, pears, & bananas	4½ oz	22	90
apricots w/pears & applesauce	4½ oz	17	70
bananas w/pears & applesauce	4½ oz	22	90
bartlett pears & pineapple	4½ oz	18	70
Fruit Dessert	4½ oz	20	80
Island Fruits	4½ oz	22	90
pears & applesauce	4½ oz	18	70
plums w/rice	4½ oz	26	110
prunes w/pears	4½ oz	30	120
Juice			
Juice Plus	4 fl oz	19	80
Main Courses			
beef & egg noodles w/vegetables	4½ oz	12	90
Beef Dinner Supreme	4½ oz	12	120
chicken & rice w/vegetables	4½ oz	13	80
chicken noodle w/vegetables	4½ oz	14	90
macaroni, tomato, & beef	4½ oz	13	90
Turkey Dinner Supreme	4½ oz	11	110
turkey rice w/vegetables	4½ oz	12	70

	Portion	Carbohydrates (g)	Total Calories
vegetable beef	4½ oz	12	90
vegetable chicken	4½ oz	14	90
vegetable ham	4½ oz	12	90
vegetable lamb	4½ oz	13	90
Vegetables			
creamed corn	4½ oz	20	90
garden vegetables	4½ oz	11	60
mixed vegetables	4½ oz	12	50
peas & carrots	4½ oz	11	60
STAGE 3			
Custard			
banana	7½ oz	43	200
vanilla	7½ oz	37	210
Fruit & Dairy			
cottage cheese w/pineapple	7½ oz	40	190
mixed fruit & yogurt	7½ oz	40	170
peaches & yogurt	7½ oz	41	190
Fruit & Fruit Dishes			
apples & grapes	7½ oz	44	190
apples & strawberries	7½ oz	40	160
applesauce	7½ oz	24	100
applesauce & bananas	7½ oz	26	110
applesauce & cherries	7½ oz	28	110
apples, mandarin oranges, & bananas	7½ oz	37	150
apples, peaches, & strawberries	7½ oz	40	160
apples, pears, & bananas	7½ oz	40	160
apricots w/pears & apples	7½ oz	29	120
bananas w/pears & apples	7½ oz	38	160
bartlett pears	7½ oz	26	110
bartlett pears & pineapple	7½ oz	30	120
Fruit Dessert	7½ oz	32	130
Island Fruits	7½ oz	37	150
peaches	7½ oz	37	150
Main Courses & Dinners			
beef & egg noodles w/vegetables	7½ oz	23	150
Beef Dinner Supreme	7½ oz	21	180
chicken noodles w/vegetables	7½ oz	23	140
macaroni, tomato, & beef	7½ oz	23	150
spaghetti, tomato, & beef	7½ oz	26	170
Turkey Dinner Supreme	7½ oz	24	190
turkey rice w/vegetables	7½ oz	20	130
vegetable bacon	7½ oz	22	180
vegetable beef	7½ oz	23	150

	Portion	Carbohydrates (g)	Total Calories
vegetable chicken	7½ oz	20	140
vegetable lamb	7½ oz	22	140
Vegetables			
carrots	7½ oz	14	60
green beans	7½ oz	13	60
mixed vegetables	7½ oz	20	90
sweet potatoes	7½ oz	27	120
UNSTAGED			
Juices			
apple	4 fl oz	14	60
apple banana	4.2 fl oz	14	60
apple cherry	4.2 fl oz	12	50
apple cranberry	4.2 fl oz	14	60
apple grape	4.2 fl oz	14	60
apple pear	4.2 fl oz	14	60
mixed fruit	4.2 fl oz	15	60
orange	4.2 fl oz	14	60
pear	4 fl oz	14	60
tropical blend	4 fl oz	17	70
TABLE TIME			
Main Courses			
beef stew	6 oz	16	140
pasta squares in meat sauce	6 oz	19	140
spaghetti rings in meat sauce	6 oz	22	160
vegetable stew w/chicken	6 oz	23	190
Soups			
Hearty chicken w/stars	6 oz	20	180
Hearty vegetable	6 oz	16	70
Gerber			
BAKED GOODS			
animal crackers	4	8	50
animal-shaped cookies	2	9	60
arrowroot cookies	2	8	50
pretzels	2	10	50
Toddler Biter biscuits	1	9	50
vanilla number cookies	4	8	60
zwieback toast	2	10	60
CHUNKY PRODUCTS			
beef & egg noodles w/vegetables	6 oz	16	130
Homestyle noodles & beef	6 oz	18	150
macaroni alphabets w/beef & tomato sauce	6¼ oz	20	130
noodles & chicken w/carrots & peas	6 oz	15	100

	Portion	Carbohydrates (g)	Total Calories
potatoes & ham	6 oz	15	110
rice w/beef & tomato sauce	6¼ oz	20	150
saucy rice w/chicken	6 oz	17	110
spaghetti tomato sauce & beef	6¼ oz	22	160
vegetables & beef	6¼ oz	17	140
vegetables & chicken	6¼ oz	17	140
vegetables & ham	6¼ oz	15	120
vegetables & turkey	6¼ oz	17	110
DRY CEREALS, READY-TO-SERVE			
barley	½ oz dry	11	60
	½ oz dry + 2.4 fl oz milk	14	110
high protein	½ oz dry	6	50
	½ oz dry + 2.4 fl oz milk	9	100
w/apple & orange	½ oz dry	8	60
	½ oz dry + 2.4 fl oz milk	11	100
mixed	½ oz dry	10	50
	½ oz dry + 2.4 fl oz milk	13	100
w/banana	½ oz dry	11	60
	½ oz dry + 2.4 fl oz milk	14	100
oatmeal	½ oz dry	9	50
	½ oz dry + 2.4 fl oz milk	12	100
w/banana	½ oz dry	10	60
	½ oz dry + 2.4 fl oz milk	13	100
rice	½ oz dry	11	60
	½ oz dry + 2.4 fl oz milk	14	100
w/banana	½ oz dry	11	60
	½ oz dry + 2.4 fl oz milk	14	100
STRAINED FOODS			
Cereals w/Fruit			
mixed w/applesauce & bananas	4½ oz	22	100
oatmeal w/applesauce & bananas	4½ oz	21	100
rice w/applesauce & bananas	4½ oz	23	100
Desserts			
banana apple	4½ oz	21	90
cherry vanilla pudding	4½ oz	21	90
chocolate custard pudding	4½ oz	21	110

	Portion	Carbohydrates (g)	Total Calories
Dutch apple	4½ oz	21	100
fruit	4½ oz	22	100
Hawaiian Delight	4½ oz	25	120
orange pudding	4½ oz	24	110
peach cobbler	4½ oz	23	100
vanilla custard pudding	4½ oz	22	100
Dinners, Regular			
beef egg noodle	4½ oz	12	90
cereal egg yolk bacon	4½ oz	10	100
chicken noodle	4½ oz	12	80
cream of chicken soup	4½ oz	11	70
macaroni cheese	4½ oz	12	90
macaroni tomato beef	4½ oz	12	80
turkey rice	4½ oz	10	80
vegetable bacon	4½ oz	11	100
vegetable beef	4½ oz	11	80
vegetable chicken	4½ oz	12	80
vegetable ham	4½ oz	11	80
vegetable lamb	4½ oz	10	90
vegetable liver	4½ oz	11	60
vegetable turkey	4½ oz	10	70
Dinners, High in Meat			
beef w/vegetables	4½ oz	8	120
chicken w/vegetables	4½ oz	8	140
ham w/vegetables	4½ oz	9	100
turkey w/vegetables	4½ oz	8	130
veal w/vegetables	4½ oz	9	100
Fruit & Tropical Fruit			
apple blueberry	4½ oz	14	60
applesauce	4½ oz	14	60
applesauce apricot	4½ oz	15	70
applesauce w/pineapple	4½ oz	14	60
apricots w/tapioca	4½ oz	20	90
bananas w/pineapple & tapioca	4½ oz	15	70
bananas w/tapioca	4½ oz	24	100
guava w/tapioca	4½ oz	20	90
mango w/tapioca	4½ oz	21	90
papaya w/tapioca	4½ oz	19	80
peaches	4½ oz	19	90
pear pineapple	4½ oz	16	80
pears	4½ oz	16	80
plums w/tapioca	4½ oz	22	100
prunes w/tapioca	4½ oz	21	100
Tropical Fruit Medley	4½ oz	19	80
Juices			
apple	4.2 oz	15	60
apple apricot	4.2 oz	15	60

	Portion	Carbohydrates (g)	Total Calories
apple banana	4.2 oz	16	70
apple cherry	4.2 oz	15	60
apple grape	4.2 oz	15	60
apple peach	4.2 oz	14	60
apple pineapple	4.2 oz	15	60
apple plum	4.2 oz	15	60
apple prune	4.2 oz	17	70
mixed fruit	4.2 oz	15	70
orange	4.2 oz	14	70
orange apple	4.2 oz	14	70
pear	4.2 oz	16	60

Meats & Egg Yolks

beef	3½ oz	0	100
beef liver	3½ oz	3	100
chicken	3½ oz	1	140
egg yolks	3½ oz	1	190
ham	3½ oz	1	110
lamb	3½ oz	1	100
pork	3½ oz	0	110
turkey	3½ oz	0	130
veal	3½ oz	0	100

Vegetables

beets	4½ oz	11	50
carrots	4½ oz	7	40
creamed corn	4½ oz	17	80
creamed spinach	4½ oz	9	60
garden vegetables	4½ oz	8	50
green beans	4½ oz	8	50
mixed vegetables	4½ oz	10	50
peas	4½ oz	10	60
squash	4½ oz	8	40
sweet potatoes	4½ oz	18	80

FIRST FOODS

Fruit

applesauce	2½ oz	7	30
bananas	2½ oz	15	60
peaches	2½ oz	7	30
pears	2½ oz	11	40

Vegetables

carrots	2½ oz	5	30
green beans	2½ oz	5	20
peas	2½ oz	6	40
squash	2½ oz	4	20
sweet potatoes	2½ oz	11	50

	Portion	Carbohydrates (g)	Total Calories
JUNIOR FOODS			
Cereals w/Fruit			
mixed w/applesauce & bananas	7½ oz	36	170
oatmeal w/applesauce & bananas	7½ oz	32	160
rice w/mixed fruit	7½ oz	39	170
Desserts			
banana apple	7½ oz	34	150
cherry vanilla pudding	7½ oz	35	150
Dutch apple	7½ oz	36	160
fruit	7½ oz	38	160
Hawaiian Delight	7½ oz	42	190
peach cobbler	7½ oz	38	160
vanilla custard pudding	7½ oz	38	190
Dinners, Regular			
beef egg noodle	7½ oz	19	140
cnicken noodle	7½ oz	18	120
macaroni tomato beef	7½ oz	22	130
spaghetti tomato sauce beef	7½ oz	25	140
split peas ham	7½ oz	24	150
turkey rice	7½ oz	17	120
vegetable bacon	7½ oz	21	180
vegetable beef	7½ oz	20	140
vegetable chicken	7½ oz	18	120
vegetable ham	7½ oz	20	140
vegetable lamb	7½ oz	19	140
vegetable turkey	7½ oz	19	120
Dinners, High in Meat			
beef w/vegetables	4½ oz	10	130
chicken w/vegetables	4½ oz	8	130
ham w/vegetables	4½ oz	10	110
turkey w/vegetables	4½ oz	9	140
veal w/vegetables	4½ oz	10	110
Fruit			
apple blueberry	7½ oz	24	110
applesauce	7½ oz	23	100
applesauce apricot	7½ oz	24	110
apricots w/tapioca	7½ oz	36	160
bananas w/pineapple & tapioca	7½ oz	25	110
bananas w/tapioca	7½ oz	39	160
peaches	7½ oz	32	140
pear pineapple	7½ oz	26	120
pears	7½ oz	27	120
plums w/tapioca	7½ oz	37	160

	Portion	Carbohydrates (g)	Total Calories
Meats			
beef	3½ oz	1	110
chicken	3½ oz	0	140
ham	3½ oz	0	120
lamb	3½ oz	0	100
turkey	3½ oz	0	130
veal	3½ oz	0	100
Vegetables			
carrots	7½ oz	12	60
creamed corn	7½ oz	27	130
creamed green beans	7½ oz	20	100
mixed vegetables	7½ oz	17	90
peas	7½ oz	20	110
squash	7½ oz	13	70
sweet potatoes	7½ oz	30	140
TODDLER FOODS			
Cereals			
Toasted Oat Rings	½ oz dry	10	60
	½ oz dry + 2.7 fl oz milk	14	110
Juices			
apple	4 oz	15	60
apple cherry	4 oz	15	60
apple grape	4 oz	15	60
apple & berry	4 oz	15	60
apple pear	4 oz	14	60
Fruits-A-Plenty	4 oz	15	60
Fruits of the Sun	4 oz	15	60
mixed fruit	4 oz	14	60
pear	4 oz	15	60
Meat & Poultry Sticks			
chicken	2½ oz	1	120
meat	2½ oz	1	110
turkey	2½ oz	1	120
Health Valley			
instant brown rice cereal	½ oz or 2 T	10	60
sprouted cereal w/bananas	⅓ oz or 2 T	11	50
Nabisco			
zwieback teething toast	2	10	60

❑ **JAMS & JELLIES** *See* FRUIT SPREADS

	Portion	Carbohydrates (g)	Total Calories

❑ **JUICE, FROZEN** *See* DESSERTS, FROZEN

❑ **JUICES & JUICE DRINKS**
See BEVERAGES

❑ **LAMB, VEAL,
& MISCELLANEOUS MEATS**

Lamb, Cooked

Lamb muscle meat (chops, leg, ribs) contains virtually no carbohydrates.

Veal, Cooked

Veal muscle meat (cutlets, scallopini, ribs) contains virtually no carbohydrates.

Other Meats

Such other meats as alligator, armadillo, frog legs, goat, rabbit, venison, & whale contain virtually no carbohydrates.

❑ **LEGUMES & LEGUME PRODUCTS**

Beans

	Portion	Carbohydrates (g)	Total Calories
adzuki			
boiled	½ c	28	147
canned, sweetened	½ c	81	351
yokan (sugar & bean confection)	1½ oz	9	36
black, boiled	½ c	20	113
black turtle soup			
boiled	1 c	45	241
canned	½ c	20	109
broad			
boiled	½ c	17	93
canned, solids & liquids	½ c	16	91
cannellini *See* kidney, *below*			
cranberry			
boiled	½ c	22	120
canned, solids & liquids	½ c	20	108
fava *See* broad, *above*			
French, boiled	½ c	21	111
garbanzo *See* chickpeas, *under* Peas & Lentils, *below*			

	Portion	Carbohydrates (g)	Total Calories
great northern			
boiled	½ c	19	104
canned, solids & liquids	½ c	28	150
green gram *See* mung, *below*			
hyacinth, boiled	½ c	20	114
kidney			
all types			
boiled	½ c	20	112
canned, solids & liquids	½ c	19	104
California red, boiled	½ c	20	109
red			
boiled	½ c	20	112
canned, solids & liquids	½ c	20	108
royal red, boiled	½ c	19	108
lima			
baby			
boiled	½ c	21	115
frozen, boiled, drained	10 oz pkg	61	326
	½ c	18	94
large			
boiled	½ c	20	108
canned, solids & liquids	½ c	18	95
frozen, boiled, drained	10 oz pkg	58	312
	½ c	16	85
long rice *See* mung, *below*			
lupins, boiled	½ c	8	98
miso *See* fermented products, *under* SOYBEANS & SOYBEAN PRODUCTS			
moth, boiled	½ c	18	103
mung			
boiled	½ c	19	107
mature seeds, sprouted			
raw	½ c	3	16
	12 oz pkg	20	102
boiled, drained	½ c	3	13
canned, drained	½ c	1	8
stir-fried	½ c	7	31
long rice, dehydrated, prepared from mung bean starch	½ c	60	246
mungo, boiled	½ c	17	95
natto *See* fermented products, *under* SOYBEANS & SOYBEAN PRODUCTS			
navy, canned, solids & liquids	½ c	27	148
okara *See* tofu: okara, *under* SOYBEANS & SOYBEAN PRODUCTS			
pink, boiled	½ c	23	125
pinto			
boiled	½ c	22	117
canned, solids & liquids	½ c	17	93
frozen, boiled, drained	10 oz pkg	88	460
Roman *See* cranberry, *above*			
shellie *See* beans, shellie, *under* VEGETABLES, PLAIN & PREPARED			

	Portion	Carbohydrates (g)	Total Calories
small white, boiled	½ c	23	127
snap *See* beans, snap, *under* VEGETABLES, PLAIN & PREPARED			
soybeans *See* SOYBEANS & SOYBEAN PRODUCTS			
tempeh *See* fermented products, *under* SOYBEANS & SOYBEAN PRODUCTS			
white			
boiled	½ c	23	125
canned, solids & liquids	½ c	29	153
winged			
raw	½ c	38	372
boiled	½ c	13	126
winged bean leaves, raw	3½ oz	14	74
winged bean tuber, raw	3½ oz	28	159
yardlong			
raw	½ c	52	292
boiled	½ c	18	102
yellow, boiled	½ c	22	126
yokan *See* adzuki, *above*			

Peas & Lentils

	Portion	Carbohydrates (g)	Total Calories
Bengal gram *See* chickpeas, *below*			
black-eyed *See* cowpeas, common, *below*			
chickpeas			
boiled	½ c	22	134
canned, solids & liquids	½ c	27	143
cowpeas, catjang, boiled	½ c	17	100
cowpeas, common			
boiled	½ c	18	100
canned, plain, solids & liquids	½ c	16	92
cowpeas, leafy tips			
raw	1 c	2	10
boiled, drained	½ c	1	6
cowpeas, young pods w/seeds			
raw	1 pod = 0.4 oz	1	5
boiled, drained	½ c	3	16
crowder peas *See* cowpeas, common, *above*			
golden gram *See* chickpeas, *above*			
lentils, boiled	½ c	20	115
lentils, sprouted			
raw	½ c	8	40
stir-fried	3½ oz	21	101
pigeon peas			
raw	½ c	64	350
boiled	½ c	20	102
red gram *See* pigeon peas, *above*			
southern peas *See* cowpeas, common, *above*			
split peas, boiled	½ c	21	116

	Portion	Carbohydrates (g)	Total Calories
Prepared Bean Dishes			
baked beans			
canned			
plain or vegetarian	½ c	26	118
w/beef	½ c	22	161
w/franks	½ c	20	182
w/pork	½ c	25	133
w/pork & sweet sauce	½ c	26	140
w/pork & tomato sauce	½ c	24	123
homemade	½ c	27	190
chili w/beans, canned	½ c	15	144
cowpeas, common, canned, w/pork	½ c	20	99
falafel	0.6 oz	5	57
	1.8 oz	16	170
hummus	1 c	50	420
refried beans, canned	½ c	23	134
• BRAND NAME			
Armour Star			
chili			
w/beans	7½ oz	27	390
w/out beans	7½ oz	14	380
Texas chili w/beans	7½ oz	22	370
Arrowhead Mills			
adzuki beans	2 oz	35	190
anasazi beans	2 oz	35	200
black turtle beans	2 oz	35	190
chickpeas	2 oz	35	200
kidney beans	2 oz	35	190
lentils			
green	2 oz	35	190
red	2 oz	34	195
mung beans			
dry, raw	2 oz	?	?
sprouted	1 c	7	50
pinto beans	2 oz	36	200
split peas, green	2 oz	35	200
Campbell			
barbecue beans	7⅞ oz	43	250
Home Style beans	8 oz	48	270
Old Fashioned beans in molasses & brown sugar	8 oz	49	270
pork & beans in tomato sauce	8 oz	43	240
Ranchero beans	7⅞ oz	34	220

	Portion	Carbohydrates (g)	Total Calories
Fearn			
BEAN MIXES			
bean barley stew	½ of 3½ oz box	33	180
black bean creole	½ of 3¾ oz box	35	180
lentil minestrone soup	½ of 3¾ oz box	26	160
split pea soup	½ of 3½ oz box	28	180
tri-bean casserole	½ of 3¼ oz box	29	160
VEGETARIAN MIXES			
breakfast patty	⅛ of 7.4 oz box	11	110
falafel	⅑ of 7.4 oz box	12	80
sesame burger	¼ c dry or ⅛ of 8.4 oz box	8	130
sunflower burger	¼ c dry or ⅛ of 8.4 oz box	15	120
Health Valley			
BEANS			
Boston baked, regular or no salt	4 oz	23	130
vegetarian, w/miso	4 oz	19	120
CHILI			
con carne	4 oz	12	170
mild vegetarian w/beans, regular or no salt	4 oz	18	170
spicy vegetarian w/beans			
regular	4 oz	18	170
no salt	4 oz	18	180
w/lentils, regular or low-sodium	4 oz	14	120
LENTILS			
Zesty pilaf, regular or no salt	4 oz	19	110
Joan of Arc Canned Vegetables			
blackeye peas	½ c	15	90
butter beans	½ c	18	100
chili beans	½ c	16	100
garbanzo beans	½ c	15	90
great northern beans	½ c	17	90
kidney beans			
dark red	½ c	20	110
light red	½ c	17	90
navy beans	½ c	17	100

	Portion	Carbohydrates (g)	Total Calories
pinto beans	½ c	18	100
pork & beans	½ c	23	130
small red beans	½ c	19	100
Van Camp's			
Beanee Weenee	1 c	32	326
brown sugar beans	1 c	48	284
butter beans	1 c	28	162
chili			
w/beans	1 c	21	352
w/out beans	1 c	12	412
kidney beans			
dark red	1 c	33	182
light red	1 c	33	184
New Orleans–style red	1 c	31	178
Mexican-style chili beans	1 c	36	210
pork & beans	1 c	39	216
red beans	1 c	36	194
vegetarian-style beans	1 c	39	206
Western-style beans	1 c	32	207
Wolf			
chili			
w/beans	1 c	22	345
w/out beans			
regular	1 c	16	387
extra spicy	scant c	15	363

❏ **LUNCHEON MEATS** *See* PROCESSED MEAT & POULTRY PRODUCTS

❏ **MAIN COURSES** *See* ENTREES & MAIN COURSES, CANNED & BOXED; ENTREES & MAIN COURSES, FROZEN

❏ **MARGARINE** *See* BUTTER & MARGARINE SPREADS

❏ **MARMALADE** *See* FRUIT SPREADS

❏ **MAYONNAISE** *See* SALAD DRESSINGS, MAYONNAISE, VINEGAR, & DIPS

	Portion	Carbohydrates (g)	Total Calories

❑ **MEAT** *See* BEEF, FRESH & CURED;
LAMB, VEAL, & MISCELLANEOUS MEATS;
PORK, FRESH & CURED; PROCESSED MEAT
& POULTRY PRODUCTS

❑ **MEAT PRODUCTS, SIMULATED**
See LEGUMES & LEGUME PRODUCTS;
NUTS & NUT-BASED BUTTERS, FLOURS,
MEALS, MILKS, PASTES, & POWDERS;
SOYBEANS & SOYBEAN PRODUCTS

❑ **MEAT SPREADS** *See* PROCESSED MEAT
& POULTRY PRODUCTS

❑ **MILK, MILK SUBSTITUTES, & MILK
PRODUCTS: CREAM, SOUR CREAM,
CREAM SUBSTITUTES, MILK, MILK
SUBSTITUTES, WHEY, & YOGURT**
See also Flavored Milk Beverages, *under*
BEVERAGES; CHEESE & CHEESE FOODS; DESSERT
SAUCES, SYRUPS, & TOPPINGS

Cream & Sour Cream

CREAM

	Portion	Carbohydrates (g)	Total Calories
half & half	1 T	1	20
	1 c	10	315
light	1 T	1	29
	1 c	9	469
medium (25% fat)	1 T	1	37
	1 c	8	583
whipping			
light	1 T	tr	44
	1 c or about 2 c whipped	7	699
heavy	1 T	tr	52
	1 c or about 2 c whipped	7	821

	Portion	Carbohydrates (g)	Total Calories
SOUR CREAM			
cultured	1 T	1	26
	1 c	10	493
half & half, cultured	1 T	1	20

Cream & Sour Cream Substitutes

coffee whitener, nondairy			
liquid, frozen, containing hy-	½ fl oz	2	20
drogenated vegetable oil &	½ c	14	163
soy protein			
liquid, frozen, containing	½ fl oz	2	20
lauric acid oil & sodium	½ c	14	164
caseinate			
powdered, containing lauric	1 t	1	11
acid oil & sodium caseinate			
imitation sour cream, nondairy,	1 oz	2	59
cultured, containing lauric	1 c	15	479
acid oil & sodium caseinate			
sour dressing, nonbutterfat,	1 T	1	21
cultured (made by combin-	1 c	11	417
ing fats or oils other than			
milk fat w/milk solids)			

Milk, Cows'

FRESH			
whole			
3.7% fat, pasteurized or raw	1 c	11	157
low-sodium	1 c	11	149
low-fat			
2% fat	1 c	12	121
2% fat, nonfat milk solids	1 c	12	125
added			
2% fat, protein-fortified	1 c	14	137
1% fat	1 c	12	102
1% fat, nonfat milk solids	1 c	12	104
added			
1% fat, protein-fortified	1 c	14	119
skim	1 c	12	86
skim, nonfat milk solids added	1 c	12	90
skim, protein-fortified	1 c	14	100
buttermilk, cultured	1 c	12	99

CONDENSED & EVAPORATED			
condensed, sweetened, canned	1 oz	21	123
	1 c	166	982

	Portion	Carbohydrates (g)	Total Calories
evaporated, canned			
whole	1 oz	3	42
	½ c	13	169
skim	1 fl oz	4	25
	½ c	14	99
DRY			
whole	¼ c	12	159
	1 c	49	635
nonfat			
regular	¼ c	16	109
	1 c	62	435
calcium-reduced	1 oz	15	100
instant	3.2 oz	47	326
	1 c	35	244
buttermilk, sweet cream	1 T	3	25
	1 c	59	464

Milk, Other

	Portion	Carbohydrates (g)	Total Calories
goat	1 c	11	168
human	1 oz	2	21
Indian buffalo	1 c	13	236
sheep	1 c	13	264

Milk Substitutes

	Portion	Carbohydrates (g)	Total Calories
filled (made by blending hydrogenated vegetable oils w/milk solids)	1 c	12	154
filled, w/lauric acid oil (made by combining milk solids w/fats or oils other than milk fat)	1 c	12	153
imitation, containing blend of hydrogenated vegetable oils	1 c	15	150
imitation, containing lauric acid	1 c	15	150

Whey

	Portion	Carbohydrates (g)	Total Calories
acid			
dry	1 T	2	10
fluid	1 c	13	59
sweet			
dry	1 T	6	26
fluid	1 c	13	66

	Portion	Carbohydrates (g)	Total Calories

Yogurt

plain
8 g protein	1 c	11	139
low-fat, 12 g protein	1 c	16	144
skim milk, 13 g protein	1 c	17	127
coffee & vanilla varieties, low-fat, 11 g protein	1 c	31	194

fruit varieties, low-fat
9 g protein	1 c	42	225
10 g protein	1 c	43	231
11 g protein	1 c	42	239

▪ BRAND NAME

Colombo Yogurt
LITE

plain	8 oz	17	110
strawberry	8 oz	42	200
vanilla	8 oz	30	160

WHOLE MILK

plain	8 oz	13	150
banana strawberry	8 oz	38	235
blueberry	8 oz	38	250
French vanilla	8 oz	29	210
peach	8 oz	37	230
strawberry	8 oz	36	230
strawberry vanilla	8 oz	45	260

Friendship
buttermilk, low-fat (1½% milk fat)	1 c	12	120
Lite Delite low-fat sour cream	2 T	2	35
sour cream	2 T	1	55

yogurt
regular (3½% milk fat), plain	1 c	15	170

low-fat (1½% milk fat)
vanilla & coffee	1 c	35	210
w/fruit	1 c	44	230

Land O'Lakes
buttermilk	8 fl oz	12	100
Flash instant, nonfat, reconstituted dry milk	8 fl oz	12	80
Gourmet heavy whipping cream	1 T	<1	60
half & half	1 T	1	20

	Portion	Carbohydrates (g)	Total Calories
milk			
homogenized	8 fl oz	11	150
low-fat (2%)	8 fl oz	11	120
low-fat (1%)	8 fl oz	12	100
skim	8 fl oz	12	90
sour cream	1 T	1	25
whipping cream	1 T	<1	45
La Yogurt			
plain	6 oz	12	130
Rich's Nondairy Creamers			
Coffee Rich	½ oz	2	22
Poly Rich	½ oz	2	22
Richwhip			
liquid	¼ oz or 1 fl oz whipped	1	20
pressurized	¼ oz	1	20
prewhipped	1 T whipped	1	12
Whitney's Yogurt			
plain	6 oz	13	150
apples & raisins	6 oz	11	200
blueberry	6 oz	33	200
boysenberry	6 oz	33	200
cherry	6 oz	33	200
coffee	6 oz	28	200
lemon	6 oz	28	200
peach	6 oz	33	200
piña colada	6 oz	33	210
raspberry	6 oz	33	200
strawberry	6 oz	33	200
strawberry banana	6 oz	33	200
tropical fruits	6 oz	33	200
vanilla	6 oz	28	200
wild berries	6 oz	33	200

□ **MOLASSES** *See* SUGARS & SWEETENERS

□ **MUFFINS** *See* BREADS, ROLLS, BISCUITS, & MUFFINS

□ **NOODLES & PASTA, PLAIN**

Noodles

chow funn, dry (Oriental wheat noodles)	1 oz	21	102

	Portion	Carbohydrates (g)	Total Calories
chow mein, canned	1 c	26	220
egg, enriched, cooked	1 c	37	200
Japanese style, seasoned *See* Nissin, *under* SOUPS, PREPARED			
rice, dry	1 oz	23	130
saimin, dry (Oriental wheat noodles)	1 oz	21	95
soba, dry (Oriental buckwheat noodles)	1 oz	20	99

Pasta

	Portion	Carbohydrates (g)	Total Calories
macaroni, enriched, cooked (cut lengths, elbows, shells)			
firm stage, hot	1 c	39	190
tender stage			
cold	1 c	24	115
hot	1 c	32	155
prepared & seasoned pasta dishes *See* DINNERS, FROZEN; ENTREES & MAIN COURSES, CANNED & BOXED; ENTREES & MAIN COURSES, FROZEN			
spaghetti, enriched, cooked			
firm stage, hot	1 c	39	190
tender stage, hot	1 c	32	155

• BRAND NAME

	Portion	Carbohydrates (g)	Total Calories
Health Valley			
elbows, whole-wheat or whole-wheat w/4 vegetables	2 oz dry	39	202
lasagna, whole-wheat	2 oz dry	39	200
spaghetti: whole-wheat, whole-wheat amaranth, or whole-wheat w/spinach	2 oz dry	40	200
spinach lasagna, whole-wheat	2 oz dry	39	170
Mueller's			
egg noodles	2 oz dry	40	220
Golden Rich egg noodles	2 oz dry	39	220
lasagna	2 oz dry	42	210
spaghetti & macaroni	2 oz dry	42	210
tricolor twists	2 oz dry	43	210
Prince			
egg noodles	3½ oz dry	73	380
macaroni & spaghetti	3½ oz dry	76	370
Superoni	3½ oz dry	65	360

	Portion	Carbohydrates (g)	Total Calories

❏ NUTS & NUT-BASED BUTTERS, FLOURS, MEALS, MILKS, PASTES, & POWDERS

See also SEEDS & SEED-BASED BUTTERS, FLOURS, & MEALS

	Portion	Carbohydrates (g)	Total Calories
acorn flour, full-fat	1 oz	16	142
acorns			
raw	1 oz	12	105
dried	1 oz	15	145
almond butter			
plain	1 T	3	101
honey & cinnamon	1 T	4	96
almond meal, partially defatted	1 oz	8	116
almond paste	1 oz	12	127
	1 c firmly packed	99	1,012
almond powder			
full-fat	1 oz	6	168
	1 c not packed	15	385
partially defatted	1 oz	9	112
	1 c not packed	21	255
almonds			
dried			
blanched	1 oz	5	166
	1 c whole kernels	27	850
unblanched	1 oz	6	167
	1 c whole kernels	29	837
dry roasted, unblanched	1 oz	7	167
	1 c whole kernels	33	810
oil roasted			
blanched	1 oz	5	174
	1 c whole kernels	26	870
unblanched	1 oz	5	176
	1 c whole kernels	25	970
toasted, unblanched	1 oz	7	167
beechnuts, dried	1 oz	10	164
Brazil nuts, dried, unblanched	1 oz	4	186
	1 c	18	919
butternuts, dried	1 oz	3	174
cashew butter, plain	1 T	4	94

	Portion	Carbohydrates (g)	Total Calories
cashew nuts			
dry roasted	1 oz	9	163
	1 c wholes & halves	45	787
oil roasted	1 oz	8	163
	1 c wholes & halves	37	748
chestnuts, Chinese			
raw	1 oz	14	64
boiled, steamed	1 oz	10	44
dried	1 oz	23	103
roasted	1 oz	15	68
chestnuts, European			
raw			
peeled	1 oz	13	56
unpeeled	1 oz	13	60
	1 c	66	308
boiled, steamed	1 oz	8	37
dried			
peeled	1 oz	22	105
unpeeled	1 oz	22	106
roasted	1 oz	15	70
	1 c	76	350
chestnuts, Japanese			
raw	1 oz	10	44
boiled, steamed	1 oz	4	16
dried	1 oz	23	102
	1 c	126	558
roasted	1 oz	13	57
coconut cream			
raw	1 T	1	49
	1 c	16	792
canned	1 T	2	36
	1 c	25	568
coconut meat			
raw	1.6 oz	7	159
	1 c shredded or grated	12	283
dried (desiccated)			
creamed	1 oz	6	194
sweetened, flaked, canned	4 oz	47	505
	1 c	32	341
sweetened, flaked, packaged	7 oz	95	944
	1 c	35	351
sweetened, shredded	7 oz	95	997
	1 c	44	466
toasted	1 oz	13	168
unsweetened	1 oz	7	187
coconut milk			
raw	1 T	1	35
	1 c	13	552

	Portion	Carbohydrates (g)	Total Calories
coconut milk *(cont.)*			
canned	1 T	tr	30
	1 c	6	445
frozen	1 T	1	30
	1 c	13	486
coconut water	1 T	1	3
	1 c	9	46
filberts or hazelnuts			
dried			
blanched	1 oz	5	191
unblanched	1 oz	4	179
	1 c chopped kernels	18	727
dry roasted, unblanched	1 oz	5	188
oil roasted, unblanched	1 oz	5	187
formulated nuts, wheat-based			
unflavored	1 oz	7	177
macadamia-flavored	1 oz	8	176
all other flavors	1 oz	6	184
ginkgo nuts			
raw	1 oz	11	52
canned	1 oz	6	32
	1 c	34	173
dried	1 oz	21	99
hazelnuts *See* filberts, *above*			
hickory nuts, dried	1 oz	5	187
macadamia nuts			
dried	1 oz	4	199
	1 c	18	940
oil roasted	1 oz	4	204
	1 c wholes or halves	17	962
mixed nuts (cashew nuts, almonds, filberts, & pecans)			
dry roasted, w/peanuts	1 oz	7	169
	1 c	35	814
oil roasted			
w/peanuts	1 oz	6	175
	1 c	30	876
w/out peanuts	1 oz	6	175
	1 c	32	886
peanut butter, w/added fat, sugar, & salt, chunk or smooth style	2 T	7	188
peanut flour			
defatted	1 c	21	196
low-fat	1 c	19	257
peanuts			
all types			
raw	1 oz	5	159
	1 c	24	828

	Portion	Carbohydrates (g)	Total Calories
boiled	½ c	7	102
dried	1 oz	5	161
	1 c	24	827
dry roasted	1 oz	6	164
	1 c	31	855
oil roasted	1 oz	5	163
	1 c	27	837
Spanish, oil roasted	1 oz	5	162
	1 c	26	851
Valencia, oil roasted	1 oz	5	165
	1 c	24	848
Virginia, oil roasted	1 oz	5	161
	1 c	28	826
pecan flour	1 oz	14	93
pecans			
dried	1 oz	5	190
	1 c halves	20	721
dry roasted	1 oz	6	187
oil roasted	1 oz	5	195
	1 c	18	754
pignolias See pine nuts, below			
pili nuts, dried	1 oz	1	204
	1 c	5	863
pine nuts			
pignolia, dried	1 oz	4	146
	1 T	1	51
piñon, dried	1 oz	5	161
	10 kernels	tr	6
pistachios			
dried	1 oz	7	164
	1 c	32	739
dry roasted	1 oz	8	172
	1 c	35	776
sweet chestnuts See chestnuts, European, above			
walnuts			
black, dried	1 oz	3	172
	1 c chopped	15	759
English or Persian, dried	1 oz	5	182
	1 c pieces	22	770

- ## BRAND NAME

Arrowhead Mills

peanut butter, creamy or chunky	2 T	6	190

Blue Diamond
almonds

raw, whole, unblanched	1 oz	5	173
blanched, sliced	1 oz	5	176

	Portion	Carbohydrates (g)	Total Calories
almonds *(cont.)*			
dry roasted, unsalted	1 oz	5	168
oil roasted, salted	1 oz	3	174
hazelnuts			
raw, whole, Oregon	1 oz	5	166
oil roasted, salted	1 oz	4	180
macadamia nuts, dry roasted, salted	1 oz	2	193
pistachios, dry roasted, salted, natural, California	1 oz	6	162
Erewhon			
almond butter	1 T	2	90
peanut butter, chunky or creamy, salted or unsalted	2 T	7	190
Fearn			
Brazil nut burger mix	¼ c dry or ⅛ of 7.6 oz box	9	100
Featherweight			
low-sodium peanut butter			
chunky	1 oz	2	90
creamy	1 oz	4	180
Planters			
almonds			
blanched: slivered, whole, or sliced	1 oz	6	170
dry roasted	1 oz	6	170
honey roasted	1 oz	9	170
cashews			
dry roasted, regular or un-salted	1 oz	9	230
honey roasted	1 oz	11	170
oil roasted, fancy or halves, regular or unsalted	1 oz	8	170
cashews & peanuts, honey roasted	1 oz	9	170
mixed nuts			
dry roasted			
regular	1 oz	7	160
unsalted	1 oz	7	170
oil roasted: regular, deluxe, or unsalted	1 oz	6	180
nut topping	1 oz	6	180
peanuts			
cocktail, oil roasted, regular or unsalted	1 oz	5	170
dry roasted			
regular	1 oz	6	160
unsalted	1 oz	5	170
honey roasted			
regular	1 oz	8	170
dry roasted	1 oz	7	160

	Portion	Carbohydrates (g)	Total Calories
oil roasted, salted	1 oz	5	170
redskin, oil roasted	1 oz	5	170
roasted-in-shell, salted or un-salted	1 oz	6	160
Spanish			
raw	1 oz	7	150
dry roasted	1 oz	6	160
oil roasted	1 oz	5	170
Sweet 'n Crunchy	1 oz	15	140
pecans: chips, halves, or pieces	1 oz	5	190
pistachios: dry roasted, natural, or red	1 oz	6	170
sesame nut mix, dry or oil roasted	1 oz	8	160
sunflower nuts			
dry roasted			
regular	1 oz	5	160
unsalted	1 oz	5	170
oil roasted	1 oz	5	170
Tavern Nuts	1 oz	6	170
walnuts			
black	1 oz	3	180
English: whole, halves, or pieces	1 oz	3	190
Skippy Peanut Butter			
creamy or super chunk	2 T	4	190
	1 T	2	95
Smucker's			
natural peanut butter	2 T	6	200

❑ **OILS** *See* FATS, OILS, & SHORTENINGS

❑ **OLIVES** *See* PICKLES, OLIVES, RELISHES, & CHUTNEYS

❑ **PASTA** *See* NOODLES & PASTA, PLAIN

❑ **PASTRIES** *See* DESSERTS: CAKES, PASTRIES, & PIES

❑ **PÂTÉS** *See* PROCESSED MEAT & POULTRY PRODUCTS

	Portion	Carbohydrates (g)	Total Calories

❑ **PEANUT BUTTER** *See* NUTS & NUT-
BASED BUTTERS, FLOURS, MEALS, MILKS,
PASTES, & POWDERS

❑ **PICKLES, OLIVES, RELISHES,
& CHUTNEYS**
See also peppers; sauerkraut, *under* VEGETABLES,
PLAIN & PREPARED

Chutneys

	Portion	Carbohydrates (g)	Total Calories
apple	1 T	11	41
tomato	1 T	8	31

Olives, Canned

	Portion	Carbohydrates (g)	Total Calories
green	4 medium or 3 extra large	tr	15
ripe, Mission, pitted	3 small or 2 large	tr	15

Pickles, Cucumber

	Portion	Carbohydrates (g)	Total Calories
bread & butter	4 slices	5	18
dill, whole	1 medium = about 2¼ oz	1	5
fresh-pack	2 slices = about ½ oz	3	10
kosher	1	1	7
sour	1 large	2	10
sweet	1 large	37	146
sweet & sour, sliced	1 slice	1	3
sweet gherkin, small, whole	1 = about ½ oz	5	20

Relishes

	Portion	Carbohydrates (g)	Total Calories
cranberry-orange	1 T	7	27
canned	½ c	64	246
pickle			
chow chow			
sour	1 oz	1	8
sweet	1 oz	8	32
sour	1 T	tr	3
sweet, finely chopped	1 T	5	20
strawberry	1 T	14	53
strawberry-pineapple	1 T	14	54
tomato	1 T	14	53

	Portion	Carbohydrates (g)	Total Calories
• BRAND NAME			
Claussen			
bread & butter pickle slices	1	1	4
kosher pickle slices	1	tr	1
kosher tomatoes	1	1	5
kosher whole pickles	1	1	7
no-garlic dills	1	2	12
pickle relish	1 T	3	13
sweet pickles	1	7	30
Dromedary			
pimientos, all types, drained	1 oz	2	10
Vlasic			
ONIONS			
lightly spiced cocktail onions	1 oz	1	4
PEPPERS			
hot banana pepper rings	1 oz	1	4
Mexican jalapeño peppers	1 oz	2	8
mild cherry peppers	1 oz	2	8
mild green pepperoncini	1 oz	1	4
PICKLES, CUCUMBER			
bread & butter sweet butter chips	1 oz	7	30
Half-the-Salt hamburger dill chips	1 oz	1	2
Hot & Spicy Garden Mix	1 oz	1	4
kosher baby dills	1 oz	1	4
kosher crunchy dills	1 oz	1	4
kosher dill gherkins	1 oz	1	4
refrigerated pickles			
Deli kosher dills	1 oz	1	4
dill bread & butter chunks	1 oz	6	25
Zesty crunchy dills	1 oz	1	4
RELISHES			
dill relish	1 oz	1	2
hamburg relish	1 oz	9	40
hot dog relish	1 oz	8	40
sweet relish	1 oz	8	30

❑ **PIE FILLINGS** *See* DESSERTS: CUSTARDS, GELATINS, PUDDINGS, & PIE FILLINGS

	Portion	Carbohydrates (g)	Total Calories

❑ **PIES** *See* DESSERTS: CAKES, PASTRIES, & PIES

❑ **PIZZA**

pizza, cheese	⅛ pizza (15″ diam)	39	290

▪ **BRAND NAME**

Celentano

9-slice pizza	⅑ pizza = 2.67 oz	20	157
thick crust pizza	⅓ pizza = 4.3 oz	31	238

Celeste Frozen Pizza

Canadian-style bacon	7¾ oz pizza	50	541
	¼ of 19 oz pizza	28	329
cheese	6½ oz pizza	48	497
	¼ of 17¾ oz pizza	28	317
deluxe	8¼ oz pizza	51	582
	¼ of 22¼ oz pizza	29	378
pepperoni	6¾ oz pizza	50	546
	¼ of 19 oz pizza	29	368
sausage	7½ oz pizza	49	571
	¼ of 20 oz pizza	30	376
sausage & mushroom	8½ oz pizza	51	592
	¼ of 22½ oz pizza	29	387
Suprema	9 oz pizza	54	678
	¼ of 23 oz pizza	29	381

Pepperidge Farm Croissant Pastry Pizza

cheese	1	47	490
deluxe	1	52	520
hamburger	1	43	510
pepperoni	1	52	490
sausage	1	53	540

Stouffer's French Bread Frozen Pizza

cheese	½ pkg	41	340
deluxe	½ pkg	41	430
hamburger	½ pkg	40	410

	Portion	Carbohydrates (g)	Total Calories
pepperoni	½ pkg	41	390
sausage	½ pkg	42	420
sausage & mushroom	½ pkg	44	400

❑ PORK, FRESH & CURED
See also PROCESSED MEAT & POULTRY PRODUCTS

Pork, Fresh

Retail cuts (loin, shank, leg, ribs, shoulder, arm) contain virtually no carbohydrates.

VARIETY MEATS

brains, braised	3 oz	0	117
chitterlings, simmered	3 oz	0	258
ears, simmered	1	0	183
feet, simmered	2½ oz	0	138
heart, braised	1	1	191
kidneys, braised	1 c	0	211
liver, braised	3 oz	3	141
lungs, braised	3 oz	0	84
tail, simmered	3 oz	0	336
tongue, braised	3 oz	0	230

Pork, Cured

bacon, pan-fried or roasted	3 medium slices (20 slices/lb)	tr	109
breakfast strips, cooked	3 slices (15 slices/12 oz)	tr	156
	6 oz	2	780
Canadian-style bacon, un-heated, fully cooked as purchased	2 oz	1	89
feet, pickled	1 oz	tr	58
ham, boneless			
regular (about 11% fat)			
unheated	1 oz	1	52
	1 c	4	255
roasted	3 oz	0	151
	1 c	0	249
extra lean (about 5% fat)			
unheated	1 oz	tr	37
	1 c	1	183
roasted	3 oz	1	123
	1 c	2	203

	Portion	Carbohydrates (g)	Total Calories
ham, canned			
regular (about 13% fat)			
unheated	1 oz	tr	54
	1 c	tr	266
roasted	3 oz	tr	192
	1 c	1	317
extra lean (about 4% fat)			
unheated	1 oz	0	34
	1 c	0	168
roasted	3 oz	tr	116
	1 c	1	191
ham, center slice			
country style, lean only, raw	4 oz	tr	220
	1 oz	tr	55
lean & fat, unheated, fully	4 oz	tr	229
cooked as purchased	1 oz	tr	57
ham patties			
unheated, fully cooked as purchased	2.3 oz	1	206
grilled	2 oz	1	203
ham steak, boneless, extra lean, unheated, fully cooked as purchased	2 oz	0	69
ham, whole			
lean & fat			
unheated, fully cooked as	1 oz	tr	70
purchased	1 c	tr	345
roasted	3 oz	0	207
	1 c	0	341
lean only			
unheated, fully cooked as	1 oz	tr	42
purchased	1 c	tr	206
roasted	3 oz	0	133
	1 c	0	219
salt pork, raw	1 oz	0	212
separable fat (from ham & arm picnic)			
unheated, fully cooked as purchased	1 oz	tr	164
roasted	1 oz	0	167
shoulder			
arm picnic, roasted			
lean & fat	3 oz	0	238
	1 c	0	392
lean only	3 oz	0	145
	1 c	0	238

	Portion	Carbohydrates (g)	Total Calories
blade roll, lean & fat			
unheated, fully cooked as purchased	1 oz	0	76
roasted	3 oz	tr	244

• BRAND NAME

Armour & Armour Star
BACON

1877 Canadian bacon	2 oz	1	80
lower salt bacon			
raw	1 slice = 0.3 oz	tr	38
cooked	1 slice = 0.2 oz	tr	30
sliced bacon	1 slice = 0.9 oz	0	130
thick-sliced bacon	1 slice = 1.3 oz	0	190

HAM

boneless, cooked, lower salt, 93% fat-free	1 oz	1	35
canned	3 oz	2	120
canned, chopped	3 oz	7	260
Golden Star, canned	3 oz	2	90
Speedy Cut, boneless, cooked	1 oz	1	44

Oscar Mayer

all bacon, cooked	1 slice	<1	varies
breakfast strips, raw	1 strip	tr	52
all sliced ham	1 oz	<1	varies

❏ POULTRY, FRESH & PROCESSED
See also PROCESSED MEAT & POULTRY PRODUCTS

NOTE: Values are based on the following weights as purchased with giblets & neck:

chicken	
broilers or fryers	3.33 lbs
roasting	4.56 lbs
stewing	2.93 lbs
capons	6.5 lbs

	Portion	Carbohydrates (g)	Total Calories
duck			
domesticated		4.42 lbs	
wild		2.26 lbs	
goose		8.25 lbs	
guinea		1.92 lbs	
pheasant		2.15 lbs	
quail		0.27 lb	
squab		0.67 lb	
turkey			
all classes		15.47 lbs	
fryer-roasters		7.05 lbs	
young hens		12.54 lbs	
young toms		23.06 lbs	

Chicken, Fresh

CHICKEN, BROILERS OR FRYERS

	Portion	Carbohydrates (g)	Total Calories
flesh, skin, giblets, & neck			
fried			
batter-dipped	1 chicken	93	2,987
flour-coated	1 chicken	23	1,928
roasted	1 chicken	tr	1,598
stewed	1 chicken	tr	1,625
flesh & skin			
fried			
batter-dipped	½ chicken	44	1,347
flour-coated	½ chicken	10	844
roasted	½ chicken	0	715
stewed	½ chicken	0	730
flesh only			
fried	1 c	2	307
roasted	1 c	0	266
stewed	1 c	0	248
skin only			
fried			
batter-dipped	½ chicken	44	748
flour-coated	½ chicken	5	281
roasted	½ chicken	0	254
stewed	½ chicken	0	261
giblets			
fried, flour-coated	1 c	6	402
simmered	1 c	1	228
gizzard, simmered	1 c	2	222
heart, simmered	1 c	tr	268
liver, simmered	1 c	1	219
light meat w/skin			
fried			
batter-dipped	½ chicken	18	520
flour-coated	½ chicken	2	320

	Portion	Carbohydrates (g)	Total Calories
roasted	½ chicken	0	293
stewed	½ chicken	0	302
dark meat w/skin			
fried			
batter-dipped	½ chicken	26	828
flour-coated	½ chicken	8	523
roasted	½ chicken	0	423
stewed	½ chicken	0	428
light meat w/out skin			
fried	1 c	1	268
roasted	1 c	0	242
stewed	1 c	0	223
dark meat w/out skin			
fried	1 c	4	334
roasted	1 c	0	286
stewed	1 c	0	269
back, meat & skin			
fried			
batter-dipped	½ back	12	397
flour-coated	½ back	5	238
roasted	½ back	0	159
stewed	½ back	0	158
back, meat only			
fried	½ back	3	167
roasted	½ back	0	96
stewed	½ back	0	88
breast, meat & skin			
fried			
batter-dipped	½ breast	13	364
flour-coated	½ breast	2	218
roasted	½ breast	0	193
stewed	½ breast	0	202
breast, meat only			
fried	½ breast	tr	161
roasted	½ breast	0	142
stewed	½ breast	0	144
drumstick, meat & skin			
fried			
batter-dipped	1	6	193
flour-coated	1	1	120
roasted	1	0	112
stewed	1	0	116
drumstick, meat only			
fried	1	0	82
roasted	1	0	76
stewed	1	0	78
leg (drumstick & thigh), meat & skin			
fried			
batter-dipped	1	14	431
flour-coated	1	3	285

	Portion	Carbohydrates (g)	Total Calories
leg, meat & skin *(cont.)*			
roasted	1	0	265
stewed	1	0	275
leg (drumstick & thigh), meat only			
fried	1	1	195
roasted	1	0	182
stewed	1	0	187
neck, meat & skin			
fried			
batter-dipped	1	5	172
flour-coated	1	2	119
simmered	1	0	94
neck, meat only			
fried	1	tr	50
simmered	1	0	32
thigh, meat & skin			
fried			
batter-dipped	1	8	238
flour-coated	1	9	162
roasted	1	10	153
stewed	1	10	158
thigh, meat only			
fried	1	1	113
roasted	1	0	109
stewed	1	0	107
wing, meat & skin			
fried			
batter-dipped	1	5	159
flour-coated	1	1	103
roasted	1	0	99
stewed	1	0	100
wing, meat only			
fried	1	0	42
roasted	1	0	43
stewed	1	0	43
CHICKEN, ROASTING			
flesh & skin, roasted	½ chicken	0	1,071
flesh only, roasted	1 c	0	233
giblets, simmered	1 c	1	239
light meat w/out skin, roasted	1 c	0	214
dark meat w/out skin, roasted	1 c	0	250
CHICKEN, STEWING			
flesh, skin, giblets, & neck, stewed	1 chicken	tr	1,636
flesh & skin, stewed	½ chicken	0	744
flesh only, stewed	1 c	0	332
giblets, simmered	1 c	tr	281

	Portion	Carbohydrates (g)	Total Calories
light meat w/out skin, stewed	1 c	0	298
dark meat w/out skin, stewed	1 c	0	361

CHICKEN, CAPONS

flesh, skin, giblets, & neck, roasted	1 chicken	1	3,211
flesh & skin, roasted	½ chicken	0	1,457
giblets, simmered	1 c	1	238

Duck, Fresh

DOMESTICATED

flesh & skin, roasted	½ duck	0	1,287
flesh only, roasted	½ duck	0	445

WILD

flesh & skin, raw	1 lb of ready-to-cook bird	0	505
breast, meat only, raw	½ breast	0	102

Goose, Fresh, Domesticated

flesh & skin, roasted	½ goose	0	2,362
flesh only, roasted	½ goose	0	1,406
liver, raw	1	6	125

Guinea, Fresh

flesh & skin, raw	1 lb of ready-to-cook bird	0	568
flesh only, raw	1 lb of ready-to-cook bird	0	304

Pheasant, Fresh

flesh & skin, raw	1 lb of ready-to-cook bird	0	670
flesh only, raw	1 lb of ready-to-cook bird	0	435
breast, meat only, raw	½ breast	0	243
leg, meat only, raw	1	0	143

Quail, Fresh

flesh & skin, raw	1 quail	0	210
flesh only, raw	1 quail	0	123
breast, meat only, raw	1	0	69

	Portion	Carbohydrates (g)	Total Calories
Squab (Pigeon), Fresh			
flesh only, raw	1 squab	0	239
breast, meat only, raw	1	0	135
Turkey, Fresh			
TURKEY, ALL CLASSES			
flesh, skin, giblets, & neck, roasted	1 lb of ready-to-cook bird	tr	533
	1 turkey	3	8,245
flesh & skin, roasted	1 lb of ready-to-cook bird	0	498
	½ turkey	0	3,857
flesh only, roasted	1 c	0	238
skin only, roasted	½ turkey	0	1,096
giblets, simmered	1 c	3	243
gizzard, simmered	1 c	1	236
heart, simmered	1 c	3	257
liver, simmered	1 c	5	237
neck, meat only, simmered	1	0	274
TURKEY, FRYER ROASTERS			
flesh, skin, giblets, & neck, roasted	1 lb of ready-to-cook bird	tr	429
	1 turkey	1	3,029
flesh & skin, roasted	1 lb of ready-to-cook bird	0	395
	½ turkey	0	1,392
flesh only, roasted	1 lb of ready-to-cook bird	0	292
	1 c	0	210
skin only, roasted	1 lb of ready-to-cook bird	0	102
	½ turkey	0	362
TURKEY, YOUNG HENS			
flesh, skin, giblets, & neck, roasted	1 lb of ready-to-cook bird	tr	565
	1 turkey	2	7,094
flesh & skin, roasted	½ turkey	0	3,323
TURKEY, YOUNG TOMS			
flesh, skin, giblets, & neck, roasted	1 lb of ready-to-cook bird	tr	514
	1 turkey	6	11,873
flesh & skin, roasted	½ turkey	0	5,545

	Portion	Carbohydrates (g)	Total Calories
Poultry, Processed			
gravy & turkey, frozen	5 oz	7	95
turkey patties, breaded, battered, fried	2¼ oz	10	181
	3⅓ oz	15	266
turkey roasts, boneless, frozen, seasoned, light & dark meat, roasted	0.43 lb	6	304
	1.72 lbs	24	1,213
turkey sticks, breaded, battered, fried	2¼ oz	11	178

▪ BRAND NAME

	Portion	Carbohydrates (g)	Total Calories
Armour & Armour Star			
broth-basted turkey, w/ or w/out sugar	4 oz	0	180
butter-basted turkey	4 oz	0	190
turkey roast w/gravy			
white & dark meat	3.69 oz	4	150
white meat only	3.69 oz	4	140
Land O'Lakes			
TURKEY PARTS			
breast	3 oz	0	100
drumsticks	3 oz	0	120
hindquarters roast	3 oz	0	140
thighs	3 oz	0	150
wings	3 oz	0	120
TURKEY PRODUCTS			
breast fillets w/cheese	5 oz	16	300
patties	2¼ oz	10	170
sticks	2 oz	9	150
WHOLE TURKEY			
butter-basted young turkey	3 oz	<1	140
self-basting (broth) young turkey	3 oz	<1	120
young turkey	3 oz	<1	130
Tyson			
FULLY COOKED CHICKEN			
Batter Gold	about 3½ oz	10	285
buttermilk	about 3½ oz	10	285
Delecta Delicious	about 3½ oz	13	305

	Portion	Carbohydrates (g)	Total Calories
Heat N Serve (oven ready)	about 3½ oz	12	270
Honey Stung	about 3½ oz	11	260
lightly breaded	about 3½ oz	10	255
POULTRY PRODUCTS			
breast patties	3 oz	10	240
breast strips	about 3½ oz	11	270
chicken pattie	about 3½ oz	9	275
Chick'n Cheddar	3 oz	13	260
Chick'n Chunks	3 oz = 6 pieces	13	250
Chick'n Dippers	3 oz = 4 pieces	13	250
Chick'n Sticks	3 oz = 3 pieces	14	240
Heat N Serve	about 3½ oz	10	280
Sandwich Mate	about 3½ oz	14	315
School Lunch pattie	about 3½ oz	11	290
Southern Fried Chunks	3 oz	13	250
Swiss 'n Bacon	3 oz	14	280
turkey patties	3 oz	12	220
READY-TO-COOK POULTRY			
boneless breast	about 3½ oz	0	205
Cornish & split Cornish	about 3½ oz	0	240
IQF chicken & split broilers	about 3½ oz	0	245
prebreaded marinated chicken	about 3½ oz	9	285

❏ **POULTRY SPREADS** *See* PROCESSED
MEAT & POULTRY PRODUCTS

❏ **PRESERVES** *See* FRUIT SPREADS

❏ **PROCESSED MEAT & POULTRY PRODUCTS: SAUSAGES, FRANKFURTERS, COLD CUTS, PÂTÉS, & SPREADS**
See also BEEF, FRESH & CURED; PORK, FRESH &
CURED; POULTRY, FRESH & PROCESSED

bacon & Canadian-style bacon *See* PORK, FRESH & CURED			
barbecue loaf, pork, beef	1 oz	2	49
beef sausage, smoked	1 oz	1	89
	1½ oz	1	134

	Portion	Carbohydrates (g)	Total Calories
beerwurst, beer salami			
beef	0.2 oz	tr	19
	0.8 oz	tr	75
pork	0.2 oz	tr	14
	0.8 oz	tr	55
berliner, pork, beef	1 oz	1	65
blood sausage	1 oz	tr	107
bockwurst, raw (pork, veal)	2½ oz	tr	200
	1 oz	tr	87
bologna			
beef	0.8 oz	tr	72
	1 oz	1	89
beef & pork	0.8 oz	1	73
	1 oz	1	89
pork	0.8 oz	tr	57
	1 oz	tr	70
turkey	1 oz	tr	57
bratwurst, cooked, pork	3 oz	2	256
	1 oz	1	85
braunschweiger (a liver sausage), pork	0.6 oz	1	65
	1 oz	1	102
breakfast strips *See* BEEF, FRESH & CURED; PORK, FRESH & CURED			
brotwurst, pork, beef	2½ oz	2	226
	1 oz	1	92
cheesefurter, pork, beef	1½ oz	1	141
chicken, canned, boned, w/ broth	5 oz	0	234
chicken roll, light meat	2 oz	1	90
	6 oz	4	271
chicken spread, canned	1 T	1	25
	1 oz	2	55
chorizo, pork & beef	1 oz	?	?
corned beef, braised *See* BEEF, FRESH & CURED			
corned beef, canned	1 oz	?	71
corned beef loaf, jellied	1 oz	0	46
dried beef	1 oz	tr	47
Dutch brand loaf, pork, beef	1 oz	2	68
frankfurter			
beef	2 oz	1	184
	1.6 oz	1	145
beef & pork	2 oz	1	183
	1.6 oz	1	144
chicken	1.6 oz	3	116
	1 oz	2	73
turkey	1.6 oz	1	102
	1 oz	tr	64
ham, boneless or canned *See* PORK, FRESH & CURED			
ham, chopped	1 oz	0	65
ham, chopped, canned	1 oz	tr	68

	Portion	Carbohydrates (g)	Total Calories
ham, minced	1 oz	1	75
ham & cheese loaf or roll	1 oz	tr	73
ham & cheese spread	1 T	tr	37
	1 oz	1	69
ham salad spread	1 T	2	32
	1 oz	3	61
head cheese, pork	1 oz	tr	60
honey loaf, pork, beef	1 oz	2	36
honey roll sausage, beef	1 oz	1	52
hot dog *See* frankfurter, *above*			
Italian sausage, pork			
raw	3.2 oz	1	315
	4 oz	1	391
cooked	2.3 oz	1	216
	2.9 oz	1	268
kielbasa, pork, beef	1 oz	1	88
knockwurst, pork, beef	2.4 oz	1	209
	1 oz	1	87
Lebanon bologna, beef	0.8 oz	tr	52
	1 oz	1	64
liver cheese, pork	1.3 oz	1	115
	1 oz	1	86
liver sausage (liverwurst), pork	1 oz	1	93
luncheon meat			
beef, jellied	1 oz	0	31
beef, loaved	1 oz	1	87
beef, thin-sliced	1 oz	tr	35
pork, beef	1 oz	1	100
pork, canned	1 oz	1	95
luncheon sausage, pork & beef	0.8 oz	tr	60
	1 oz	tr	74
mortadella, beef, pork	about ½ oz	tr	47
	1 oz	1	88
New England brand sausage,	0.8 oz	1	37
pork, beef	1 oz	1	46
olive loaf, pork	1 oz	3	67
pastrami			
beef	1 oz	1	99
turkey	2 oz	1	80
	8 oz	4	320
pâté			
chicken liver, canned	1 T	1	26
	1 oz	2	57
goose liver, smoked, canned	1 T	1	60
	1 oz	1	131
liver (not specified), canned	1 T	tr	41
	1 oz	tr	90
peppered loaf, pork, beef	1 oz	1	42

	Portion	Carbohydrates (g)	Total Calories
pepperoni, pork, beef	8.8 oz	7	1,248
	0.2 oz	tr	27
pickle & pimento loaf	1 oz	2	74
picnic loaf, pork, beef	1 oz	1	66
Polish sausage, pork	8 oz	4	739
	1 oz	tr	92
pork & beef sausage, fresh, cooked	about 1 oz	1	107
	about ½ oz	tr	52
pork sausage, country style, fresh, cooked	about 1 oz	tr	100
	about ½ oz	tr	48
salami			
cooked			
beef	0.8 oz	1	58
	1 oz	1	72
beef & pork	0.8 oz	1	57
	1 oz	1	71
turkey	2 oz	tr	111
	8 oz	1	446
dry or hard			
pork	0.35 oz	tr	41
	4 oz	2	460
pork, beef	0.35 oz	tr	42
	4 oz	3	472
sandwich spread			
pork, beef	1 T	2	35
	1 oz	3	67
poultry salad	1 T	1	26
	1 oz	2	57
smoked chopped beef	1 oz	1	38
smoked link sausage			
pork, grilled	2.4 oz	1	265
	about ½ oz	tr	62
pork & beef	2.4 oz	1	229
	about ½ oz	tr	54
flour & nonfat dry milk added	2.4 oz	3	182
	about ½ oz	1	43
nonfat dry milk added	2.4 oz	1	213
	about ½ oz	tr	50
Thuringer, cervelat, summer sausage: beef, pork	0.8 oz	1	80
	1 oz	1	98
turkey			
canned, boned, w/broth	5 oz	0	231
diced, light & dark, seasoned	1 oz	tr	39
	½ lb	2	313
turkey breast meat	0.7 oz	0	23
turkey ham (cured turkey thigh meat)	2 oz	tr	73
	8 oz	1	291

	Portion	Carbohydrates (g)	Total Calories
turkey loaf, breast meat	1½ oz	0	47
	6 oz	0	187
turkey pastrami *See* pastrami: turkey, *above*			
turkey roll, light meat	1 oz	tr	42
turkey roll, light & dark meat	1 oz	1	42
Vienna sausage, canned, beef & pork	0.6 oz	tr	45

▪ BRAND NAME

Armour & Armour Star
FRANKFURTERS

lower salt Jumbo & Jumbo Beef	2 oz	2	170
regular Jumbo & Jumbo Beef	2 oz	2	190
turkey	2 oz	3	110

LUNCHEON MEATS

bologna or beef bologna			
regular	1 oz	1	100
lower salt	1 oz	1	90
salami, regular or lower salt, cooked	1 oz	2	80
spiced luncheon meat			
regular	3 oz	5	280
w/chicken	3 oz	7	280
turkey bologna	4 oz	6	220
turkey cotto salami	4 oz	4	180
turkey ham	4 oz	2	140
turkey meat loaf	3 oz	8	160
turkey pastrami	4 oz	1	140
turkey roll, Magic Slice, cooked, white or white & dark	3 oz	0	120

MEAT PRODUCTS, CANNED

corned beef hash	1½ oz	17	390
deviled ham	1½ oz	0	110
Deviled Treet	1½ oz	1	120
potted meat	1½ oz	1	80
roast beef hash	7½ oz	20	350
sliced dried beef	1 oz	1	60
sloppy joes, beef	about 7½ oz	28	390
smoked Vienna sausage	2 oz	1	180
Vienna sausage in beef stock	2 oz	1	180

	Portion	Carbohydrates (g)	Total Calories
SAUSAGES			
sausage links, regular or lower salt, uncooked	1 oz	1	110
sausage patties, regular or lower salt, uncooked	1½ oz	1	160
sausage rolls, regular or lower salt, uncooked	1 oz	1	110
Health Valley			
bologna			
beef, sliced	3½ oz	2	310
chicken	3½ oz	2	300
frankfurters			
beef	3½ oz	2	288
chicken	3½ oz	2	290
turkey	3½ oz	2	238
knockwurst	3½ oz	2	280
pork, sliced, breakfast	3½ oz	0	560
salami, sliced	3½ oz	2	400
Land O'Lakes			
diced turkey, white & dark mixed	3 oz	<1	120
turkey ham	3 oz	2	100
Louis Rich			
barbecued breast of turkey	1 oz	tr	38
ground turkey	1 cooked oz	0	61
hickory smoked breast of turkey	1 oz	tr	35
oven roasted breast of turkey	1 oz	tr	36
oven roasted chicken breast	1 oz	tr	39
smoked turkey breast, sliced	¾ oz	tr	21
turkey breast	1 cooked oz	0	51
turkey franks	1 link = 1.58 oz	1	103
turkey ham	1 oz	tr	34
turkey pastrami	1 oz	tr	33
turkey salami	1 oz	tr	52
turkey smoked sausage	1 oz	tr	55
Oscar Mayer			
frankfurters, all	1	<2	varies
luncheon meats, all sliced beef & pork	1 slice	<3½	varies
sausages, all	1 link	<1	varies
smoked chicken breast	1 oz	tr	27
smoked turkey breast	0.7 oz	tr	20
spreads			
braunschweiger liver sausage	1 oz	1	95
ham & cheese	1 oz	1	66
ham salad	1 oz	4	62
sandwich	1 oz	4	67

	Portion	Carbohydrates (g)	Total Calories
Swanson			
chunk premium white chicken, canned	2½ oz	0	90
chunk-style Mixin' Chicken, canned	2½ oz	0	130
chunk white & dark chicken, canned	2½ oz	0	100
chunky chicken spread	1 oz	2	60
Tyson			
all white cooked chicken fryer meat	about 3½ oz	tr	166
breast of chicken roll, whole & diced	about 3½ oz	tr	155
chicken bologna	about 3½ oz	5	230
chicken corn dogs	about 3½ oz	28	280
chicken franks	about 3½ oz	2	285
Liberty Roll, whole or diced	about 3½ oz	tr	185
natural proportioned cooked chicken meat	about 3½ oz	tr	170

❏ **PUDDING DESSERTS, FROZEN**
See DESSERTS, FROZEN

❏ **PUDDINGS & PIE FILLINGS**
See DESSERTS: CUSTARDS, GELATINS, PUDDINGS, & PIE FILLINGS

❏ **RELISHES** *See* PICKLES, OLIVES, RELISHES, & CHUTNEYS

❏ **RICE & GRAINS, PLAIN & PREPARED**
See also VEGETABLES, PLAIN & PREPARED

	Portion	Carbohydrates (g)	Total Calories
barley, pearled, light, uncooked	1 c	158	700
bulgur, uncooked	1 c	129	600
hominy grits *See* corn grits, *under* BREAKFAST CEREALS, COLD & HOT			
popcorn *See* SNACKS			
rice			
brown, cooked, hot	1 c	50	230
white, enriched			
raw	1 c	149	670
cooked, hot	1 c	50	225

	Portion	Carbohydrates (g)	Total Calories
instant, ready-to-serve, hot	1 c	40	180
parboiled, raw	1 c	150	685
parboiled, cooked, hot	1 c	41	185

• BRAND NAME

Arrowhead Mills
PLAIN RICE & GRAINS

barley, pearled, or barley flakes	2 oz	45	200
buckwheat groats, brown or white	2 oz	41	190
bulgur wheat	2 oz	43	200
corn			
blue	2 oz	41	210
yellow	2 oz	43	210
millet	2 oz	21	90
oat flakes	2 oz	39	220
oat groats	2 oz	38	220
quinoa	2 oz	35	200
rice, brown: long, long basmati, medium, or short	2 oz	44	200
rye or rye flakes	2 oz	42	190
triticale or triticale flakes	2 oz	41	190
wheat, hard, red, winter, or soft pastry	2 oz	41	190
wheat flakes	2 oz	42	210

PREPARED RICE & GRAINS

Quick brown rice			
regular	2 oz	43	200
Spanish style	¼ of 5.65 oz pkg	30	150
vegetable herb	¼ of 5.6 oz pkg	30	150
wild rice & herbs	¼ of 5.35 oz pkg	28	140

Birds Eye International Rice Recipes

French style	3.3 oz	23	110
Italian style	3.3 oz	26	120
Spanish style	3.3 oz	24	110

Carolina Rice

extra long grain, enriched	about ½ c cooked	22	100
long grain, enriched, pre-cooked instant	about ½ c cooked	23	110

Chun King

rice mix	¼ oz	4	20

	Portion	Carbohydrates (g)	Total Calories
Fearn			
Naturfresh corn germ	¼ c or 1 oz	12	130
Naturfresh raw wheat germ	¼ c or 1 oz	13	100
Featherweight			
Spanish rice	7½ oz	30	140
Health Valley			
amaranth pilaf, regular or low-salt	4 oz	14	90
Mahatma			
long grain rice, enriched	about ½ c cooked	22	100
long grain rice, enriched, pre-cooked instant	about ½ c cooked	23	110
natural long grain rice, brown	about ½ c cooked	23	110
Minute Rice			
drumstick mix, w/salted butter	½ c	25	150
fried rice mix, w/oil	½ c	25	160
long grain & wild rice mix, w/ salted butter	½ c	25	150
rib roast mix, w/salted butter	½ c	25	150
rice, w/out salt or butter	⅔ c	27	120
Pillsbury Frozen Rice Originals			
Italian blend white rice & spinach in cheese sauce	½ c	23	170
long grain white & wild rice	½ c	23	120
Rice Jubilee	½ c	22	150
Rice Medley	½ c	21	120
rice & broccoli in flavored cheese sauce	½ c	18	120
rice pilaf	½ c	23	120
rice w/herb butter sauce	½ c	22	150
Quaker Oats			
Scotch brand medium or quick pearled barley	¼ c	36	172
Rice-A-Roni			
MICROWAVE LONG GRAIN & WILD RICE MIXES			
original flavor w/herbs & seasoning, prepared	½ c	24	140
chicken flavor & mushroom, prepared	½ c	24	140
RICE & PASTA MIXES			
beef flavor, prepared	½ c	27	170
beef flavor & mushroom, prepared	½ c	24	150
chicken & mushroom flavor, prepared	½ c	26	180
chicken flavor, prepared	½ c	28	170

	Portion	Carbohydrates (g)	Total Calories
chicken flavor & vegetables, prepared	½ c	24	140
chicken flavor/chicken broth w/ herbs, twin pack, prepared	⅔ c	35	220
fried rice w/almonds, prepared	½ c	21	140
herb & butter, prepared	½ c	22	130
rice pilaf, prepared	½ c	30	190
risotto, prepared	¾ c	32	210
Spanish rice, prepared	½ c	24	140
Stroganoff w/sour cream sauce, prepared	½ c	27	200

RICE MIXES

brown & wild rice w/mushrooms, prepared	½ c	24	180
long grain & wild rice w/herbs & seasoning, prepared	½ c	21	140
yellow rice dinner, prepared	¾ c	43	250
River			
enriched rice	about ½ c cooked	22	100
natural long grain rice, brown	about ½ c cooked	23	110
Riviana Make-It-Easy			
beef-flavored rice & vermicelli mix	⅙ of 8 oz box or about ½ c cooked	28	130
chicken-flavored rice & vermicelli mix	⅙ of 8 oz box or about ½ c cooked	28	130
Stouffer			
apple pecan rice	½ of 5⅞ oz pkg	22	130
Rice Medley	3 oz	20	110
Success			
enriched, precooked, natural long grain rice	about ½ c cooked	21	100
Van Camp's			
Golden Hominy	1 c	28	128
Spanish rice	1 c	28	150
Water Maid			
enriched rice	about ½ c cooked	22	100

❑ **ROLLS** *See* BREADS, ROLLS, BISCUITS, & MUFFINS

	Portion	Carbohydrates (g)	Total Calories

◻ SALAD DRESSINGS, MAYONNAISE, VINEGAR, & DIPS

Mayonnaise, Commercial

mayonnaise			
safflower & soybean	1 c	6	1,577
	1 T	tr	99
soybean	1 c	6	1,577
	1 T	tr	99
mayonnaise, imitation			
milk, cream	1 c	27	232
	1 T	2	15
soybean	1 c	38	556
	1 T	2	35
soybean w/out cholesterol	1 c	36	1,084
	1 T	2	68
mayonnaise-type dressing			
regular	1 c	56	916
	1 T	4	57
low-cal	1 T	1	19

Salad Dressings

bleu cheese, commercial			
regular	1 c	18	1,235
	1 T	1	77
low-cal	1 T	1	11
Caesar, commercial	1 T	1	70
coleslaw, commercial, low-cal	1 T	0	31
cooked, homemade	1 c	38	400
	1 T	2	25
French			
commercial			
regular	1 c	44	1,074
	1 T	3	67
creamy	1 T	2	70
low-cal	1 c	56	349
	1 T	4	22
homemade	1 c	8	1,388
	1 T	1	88
Green Goddess, commercial			
regular	1 T	1	68
low-cal	1 T	2	27
Italian, commercial			
regular	1 c	24	1,098
	1 T	2	69
creamy	1 T	3	52
low-cal	1 c	12	253
	1 T	1	16

	Portion	Carbohydrates (g)	Total Calories
Russian, commercial			
regular	1 c	26	1,210
	1 T	2	76
low-cal	1 c	72	368
	1 T	5	23
poppy seed	1 oz	6	121
sesame seed, commercial	1 c	21	1,086
	1 T	1	68
sweet & sour, commercial	1 T	7	29
Thousand Island, commercial			
regular	1 c	38	943
	1 T	2	59
low-cal	1 c	40	389
	1 T	3	24
vinegar & oil, homemade	1 c	6	1,122
	1 T	tr	72
vinegar (red wine) & oil, commercial	1 oz	7	103

Vinegar

cider	1 T	1	tr
distilled	1 T	1	2

▪ BRAND NAME

Featherweight
LOW-SALT DRESSINGS

Soyamaise	1 T	0	100

LOW-SALT, LOW-CAL DRESSINGS

Caesar	1 T	2	14
creamy cucumber	1 T	1	4
French	1 T	3	14
herb	1 T	1	6
Italian	1 T	1	4
New Bleu	1 T	1	4
red wine vinegar	1 T	1	6
Russian	1 T	1	6
Thousand Island	1 T	3	18
Zesty Tomato	1 T	0	2

Good Seasons Salad Dressing Mixes

bleu cheese & herbs, w/vinegar, water, & salad oil	1 T	1	80
Buttermilk Farm Style, w/whole milk & mayonnaise	1 T	1	60

	Portion	Carbohydrates (g)	Total Calories
cheese garlic, w/vinegar, water, & salad oil	1 T	1	80
cheese Italian, w/vinegar, water, & salad oil	1 T	1	80
classic herb, w/vinegar, water, & salad oil	1 T	0	80
garlic & herbs, w/vinegar, water, & salad oil	1 T	1	80
Italian, w/vinegar, water, & salad oil	1 T	1	80
lemon & herbs, w/vinegar, water, & salad oil	1 T	1	80
lite Italian, w/vinegar, water, & salad oil	1 T	1	25
no-oil Italian, w/vinegar & water	1 T	2	6
Hellman's			
Real mayonnaise	1 T	0	100
sandwich spread	1 T	2	50
tartar sauce	1 T	0	70
Land O'Lakes			
dips, flavored, dairy	2 oz	4	70
Life All Natural			
avocado dressing/dip w/tofu	½ oz	1	70
creamy salad dressing, egg-free, low-cholesterol	½ oz	2	39
garlic dressing/dip w/tofu	½ oz	1	70
mayonnaise-style dressing, egg-free, low-cholesterol	½ oz	1	71
tofu dressing/dip	½ oz	1	75
Ortega			
Acapulco Dip	1 oz	2	8
Regina			
wine vinegars, all flavors	1 fl oz	0	4

❑ **SALADS, COMMERCIALLY PREPARED**
See FAST FOODS; FRUIT, FRESH
& PROCESSED; VEGETABLES, PLAIN
& PREPARED

❑ **SAUCES, DESSERT** *See* DESSERT
SAUCES, SYRUPS, & TOPPINGS

	Portion	Carbohydrates (g)	Total Calories

❑ SAUCES, GRAVIES, & CONDIMENTS

See also FRUIT, FRESH & PROCESSED; PICKLES, OLIVES, RELISHES, & CHUTNEYS

Condiments

	Portion	Carbohydrates (g)	Total Calories
catsup	1 c	69	290
mustard, prepared, yellow	1 t	tr	5

Gravies

	Portion	Carbohydrates (g)	Total Calories
au jus			
canned	1 c	6	38
	10½ oz	7	48
dehydrated, prepared w/water	1 c	2	19
	21.7 oz	6	48
beef, canned	1 c	11	124
	10¼ oz	14	155
brown, dehydrated, prepared	1 c	2	9
w/water	9.7 oz	2	9
chicken			
canned	1 c	13	189
	10½ oz	16	236
dehydrated, prepared w/water	1 c	14	83
mushroom			
canned	1 c	13	120
	10½ oz	16	150
dehydrated, prepared w/water	1 c	14	70
onion, dehydrated, prepared w/ water	1 c	17	80
pork, dehydrated, prepared w/ water	1 c	13	76
turkey			
canned	1 c	12	122
	10½ oz	15	152
dehydrated, prepared w/water	1 c	15	87

Sauces

	Portion	Carbohydrates (g)	Total Calories
barbecue, ready-to-serve	1 c	32	188
béarnaise			
dehydrated	0.9 oz	15	90
dehydrated, prepared w/milk	1 c	18	701
& butter	13½ oz	26	1,052
cheese			
dehydrated	1.2 oz	12	158
dehydrated, prepared w/whole milk	1 c	23	307

	Portion	Carbohydrates (g)	Total Calories
curry			
dehydrated	1.2 oz	18	151
dehydrated, prepared w/whole	1 c	26	270
milk	12 oz	32	337
hollandaise, dehydrated			
w/butterfat	1.2 oz	11	187
w/butterfat, prepared w/water	1 c	14	237
	7.2 oz	11	187
w/vegetable oil	1 oz	15	93
w/vegetable oil, prepared w/	1 c	18	703
milk & butter	13½ oz	27	1,055
marinara, canned	1 c	25	171
	15½ oz	45	300
mushroom			
dehydrated	1 oz	16	99
dehydrated, prepared w/whole	1 c	24	228
milk	11.7 oz	30	285
sour cream			
dehydrated	1.2 oz	17	180
dehydrated, prepared w/whole	1 c	45	509
milk	5½ oz	23	255
soy *See* SOYBEANS & SOYBEAN PRODUCTS			
spaghetti			
canned	1 c	40	272
	15½ oz	70	479
dehydrated	0.35 oz	6	28
	1½ oz	27	118
dehydrated, w/mushrooms	0.35 oz	5	30
	1.4 oz	19	118
Stroganoff			
dehydrated	1.6 oz	27	161
dehydrated, prepared w/whole	1 c	34	271
milk & water	11.2 oz	37	292
sweet & sour			
dehydrated	2 oz	55	220
dehydrated, prepared w/water	1 c	73	294
& vinegar	8.3 oz	55	220
tamari *See* SOYBEANS & SOYBEAN PRODUCTS			
teriyaki *See* SOYBEANS & SOYBEAN PRODUCTS			
tomato, canned	½ c	9	37
Spanish style	½ c	9	40
w/herbs & cheese	½ c	13	72
w/mushrooms	½ c	10	42
w/onions	½ c	12	52

	Portion	Carbohydrates (g)	Total Calories
w/onions, green peppers, & celery	½ c	11	50
w/tomato tidbits	½ c	9	39
tomato paste & puree *See* VEGETABLES, PLAIN & PREPARED			
white			
dehydrated	1.7 oz	25	230
dehydrated, prepared w/whole	1 c	21	241
milk	23.2 oz	54	602

▪ BRAND NAME

A-1
steak sauce	1 T	3	12
Chun King			
mustard, brown	1 t	0	4
sauce/glaze mix for sweet & sour entree	3.8 oz	96	370
sweet & sour sauce	1.8 oz	14	60
Escoffier			
Sauce Diable	1 T	4	20
Sauce Robert	1 T	5	20
Franco-American Gravies			
au jus	2 oz	1	5
beef	2 oz	3	25
brown, w/onions	2 oz	4	25
chicken	2 oz	3	50
chicken giblet	2 oz	3	30
mushroom	2 oz	3	25
pork	2 oz	3	40
turkey	2 oz	3	30
Fresh Chef Sauces			
Bolognese	4 oz	13	130
pesto	4 oz	12	630
red clam	4 oz	10	90
tomato	4 oz	12	160
white clam	4 oz	5	130
Grey Poupon			
Dijon mustard	1 T	0	18
Health Valley			
Catch-Up, regular or no salt	1 T	3	16
tomato sauce, regular or no salt	4 oz	5	30
Life All Natural			
English mustard	¼ oz	tr	11
horseradish sauce	¼ fl oz	tr	7
steak sauce	½ oz	3	11

	Portion	Carbohydrates (g)	Total Calories
tartar sauce, egg-free, low-cholesterol	¼ fl oz	1	19
tomato catsup	½ oz	3	11
Worcestershire sauce	¼ oz	1	5
Open Pit Barbecue Sauce			
original flavor	1 T	6	25
hickory smoke flavor	1 T	5	25
Hot 'n Tangy flavor	1 T	5	25
Mesquite 'n Tangy flavor	1 T	6	25
Sweet 'n Tangy flavor	1 T	6	25
Ortega			
enchilada sauce, mild or hot	1 oz	3	12
green chile salsa			
mild or medium	1 oz	2	8
hot	1 oz	2	10
Picante salsa	1 oz	2	10
Ranchera salsa	1 oz	3	12
taco salsa, mild or hot	1 oz	2	10
taco sauce, mild or hot	1 oz	3	12
Western-style taco sauce	1 oz	2	8
Prego			
Al Fresco Garden tomato sauce	4 oz	12	100
Prego Plus			
w/beef sirloin & onion	4 oz	20	160
w/mushrooms & chunk	4 oz	18	130
w/sausage & green peppers	4 oz	19	170
w/veal & sliced mushrooms	4 oz	20	150
spaghetti sauce	4 oz	20	140
spaghetti sauce, meat-flavored	4 oz	21	150
Steak Supreme			
steak sauce	1 T	5	20
Tabasco			
Tabasco sauce	¼ t	tr	1
Wolf			
chili hot dog sauce	about ⅛ c	4	44

❏ SEAFOOD & SEAFOOD PRODUCTS

See also DINNERS, FROZEN;
ENTREES & MAIN COURSES, FROZEN

Finfish

ahi *See* tuna: yellowfin, *below*			
aku *See* tuna: skipjack, *below*			
anchovy, European			
raw	3 oz	0	111
canned in oil, drained solids	5	0	42

	Portion	Carbohydrates (g)	Total Calories
bass, freshwater			
mixed species, raw	3 oz	0	97
striped, raw	3 oz	0	82
bluefish, raw	3 oz	0	105
burbot, raw	3 oz	0	76
butterfish, raw	3 oz	0	124
carp			
raw	3 oz	0	108
baked, broiled, microwaved	3 oz	0	138
catfish			
channel			
raw	3 oz	0	99
breaded & fried	3 oz	7	194
ocean *See* wolffish, *below*			
chub *See* cisco: smoked, *below*			
cisco			
raw	3 oz	0	84
smoked	1 oz	0	50
	3 oz	0	151
cod			
Atlantic			
raw	3 oz	0	70
baked, broiled, microwaved	3 oz	0	89
canned, solids & liquids	3 oz	0	89
dried & salted	1 oz	0	81
	3 oz	0	246
Pacific, raw	3 oz	0	70
croaker, Atlantic			
raw	3 oz	0	89
breaded & fried	3 oz	6	188
cusk, raw	3 oz	0	74
dogfish *See* shark, *below*			
dolphin fish, raw	3 oz	0	73
drum, freshwater, raw	3 oz	0	101
eel, mixed species			
raw	3 oz	0	156
baked, broiled, microwaved	3 oz	0	200
flatfish			
raw	3 oz	0	78
baked, broiled, microwaved	3 oz	0	99
flounder *See* flatfish, *above*			
grouper, mixed species			
raw	3 oz	0	78
baked, broiled, microwaved	3 oz	0	100
haddock			
raw	3 oz	0	74
baked, broiled, microwaved	3 oz	0	95
smoked	1 oz	0	33
	3 oz	0	99
hake *See* whiting, *below*			

	Portion	Carbohydrates (g)	Total Calories
halibut			
Atlantic or Pacific			
raw	3 oz	0	93
baked, broiled, microwaved	3 oz	0	119
Greenland, raw	3 oz	0	158
herring			
Atlantic			
raw	3 oz	0	134
baked, broiled, microwaved	3 oz	0	172
canned *See* sardine: Atlantic, *below*			
kippered	1.4 oz	0	87
pickled	½ oz	1	39
lake *See* cisco, *above*			
Pacific, raw	3 oz	0	166
jack *See* mackerel: jack, *below*			
ling, raw	3 oz	0	74
lingcod, raw	3 oz	0	72
lox *See* salmon: chinook, smoked, *below*			
mackerel			
Atlantic			
raw	3 oz	0	174
baked, broiled, microwaved	3 oz	0	223
jack, canned, drained solids	1 c	0	296
king, raw	3 oz	0	89
Pacific & jack, mixed species, raw	3 oz	0	133
Spanish			
raw	3 oz	0	118
baked, broiled, microwaved	3 oz	0	134
mahimahi *See* dolphin fish, *above*			
milkfish, raw	3 oz	0	126
monkfish, raw	3 oz	0	64
mullet, striped			
raw	3 oz	0	99
baked, broiled, microwaved	3 oz	0	127
ocean perch, Atlantic			
raw	3 oz	0	80
baked, broiled, microwaved	3 oz	0	103
perch, mixed species			
raw	3 oz	0	77
baked, broiled, microwaved	3 oz	0	99
pike			
northern			
raw	3 oz	0	75
baked, broiled, microwaved	3 oz	0	96
walleye, raw	3 oz	0	79
pollock			
Atlantic, raw	3 oz	0	78
walleye			
raw	3 oz	0	68
baked, broiled, microwaved	3 oz	0	96

	Portion	Carbohydrates (g)	Total Calories
pompano, Florida			
raw	3 oz	0	140
baked, broiled, microwaved	3 oz	0	179
porgy See scup, below			
pout, ocean, raw	3 oz	0	67
redfish See ocean perch, above			
rockfish, Pacific, mixed species			
raw	3 oz	0	80
baked, broiled, microwaved	3 oz	0	103
roughy, orange, raw	3 oz	0	107
sablefish			
raw	3 oz	0	166
smoked	1 oz	0	72
salmon			
Atlantic, raw	3 oz	0	121
chinook			
raw	3 oz	0	153
smoked	1 oz	0	33
	3 oz	0	99
chum			
raw	3 oz	0	102
canned, drained solids w/	3 oz	0	120
bone	13 oz	0	521
coho			
raw	3 oz	0	124
boiled, poached, steamed	3 oz	0	157
pink			
raw	3 oz	0	99
canned, solids w/bone & liq-	3 oz	0	118
uid	16 oz	0	631
red See sockeye, below			
sockeye			
raw	3 oz	0	143
baked, broiled, microwaved	3 oz	0	183
canned, drained solids w/	3 oz	0	130
bone	13 oz	0	566
sardine			
Atlantic, canned in oil,	2 sardines =	0	50
drained solids w/bone	0.8 oz		
	3.2 oz	0	192
Pacific, canned in tomato	1 sardine =	0	68
sauce, drained solids w/	1.3 oz		
bone	13 oz	0	658
scrod See cod: Atlantic, above			
scup, raw	3 oz	0	89

	Portion	Carbohydrates (g)	Total Calories
sea bass, mixed species			
raw	3 oz	0	82
baked, broiled, microwaved	3 oz	0	105
sea trout, mixed species, raw	3 oz	0	88
shad, American, raw	3 oz	0	167
shark, mixed species			
raw	3 oz	0	111
batter-dipped & fried	3 oz	5	194
sheepshead			
raw	3 oz	0	92
baked, broiled, microwaved	3 oz	0	107
smelt, rainbow			
raw	3 oz	0	83
baked, broiled, microwaved	3 oz	0	106
snapper, mixed species			
raw	3 oz	0	85
baked, broiled, microwaved	3 oz	0	109
sole *See* flatfish, *above*			
spot, raw	3 oz	0	105
sturgeon, mixed species			
raw	3 oz	0	90
baked, broiled, microwaved	3 oz	0	115
smoked	1 oz	0	48
	3 oz	0	147
sucker, white, raw	3 oz	0	79
sunfish, pumpkinseed, raw	3 oz	0	76
swordfish			
raw	3 oz	0	103
baked, broiled, microwaved	3 oz	0	132
tilefish			
raw	3 oz	0	81
baked, broiled, microwaved	3 oz	0	125
trout			
mixed species, raw	3 oz	0	126
rainbow			
raw	3 oz	0	100
baked, broiled, microwaved	3 oz	0	129
tuna			
bluefin			
raw	3 oz	0	122
baked, broiled, microwaved	3 oz	0	157
light, canned			
in soybean oil, drained sol-	3 oz	0	169
ids	6 oz	0	339
in water, drained solids	3 oz	0	111
	5.8 oz	0	216
white, canned			
in soybean oil, drained sol-	3 oz	0	158
ids	6.3 oz	0	331
in water, drained solids	3 oz	0	116
	6.1 oz	0	234

	Portion	Carbohydrates (g)	Total Calories
skipjack, raw	3 oz	0	88
yellowfin, raw	3 oz	0	92
turbot			
domestic See **halibut: Greenland,** *above*			
European, raw	3 oz	0	81
whitefish, mixed species			
raw	3 oz	0	114
smoked	1 oz	0	30
	3 oz	0	92
whiting, mixed species			
raw	3 oz	0	77
baked, broiled, microwaved	3 oz	0	98
wolffish, Atlantic, raw	3 oz	0	82
yellowtail, mixed species, raw	3 oz	0	124

Shellfish

	Portion	Carbohydrates (g)	Total Calories
abalone, mixed species			
raw	3 oz	5	89
fried	3 oz	9	161
clams, mixed species			
raw	3 oz	2	63
	9 large (50/qt) or 20 small (110/qt)	5	133
boiled, poached, steamed	3 oz	4	126
	20 small (110/qt)	5	133
breaded & fried	3 oz	9	171
	20 small (110/qt)	19	379
canned, drained solids	3 oz	4	126
	1 c	8	236
canned, liquid	3 oz	tr	2
	1 c	tr	6
crab			
Alaska king			
raw	3 oz	0	71
	1 leg = 1 lb	0	144
boiled, poached, steamed	3 oz	0	82
	1 leg = 1 lb	0	129
blue			
raw	1 crab = ⅓ lb	tr	18
	3 oz	tr	74
boiled, poached, steamed	3 oz	0	87
	1 c not packed	0	138
canned, dry pack or drained solids of wet pack	3 oz	0	84
	1 c not packed	0	133

	Portion	Carbohydrates (g)	Total Calories
crab *(cont.)*			
Dungeness, raw	3 oz	1	73
	1 crab = 1½ lb	1	140
queen, raw	3 oz	0	76
crayfish, mixed species			
raw	3 oz	0	76
boiled, poached, steamed	3 oz	0	97
cuttlefish, mixed species, raw	3 oz	1	67
lobster, northern			
raw	3 oz	tr	77
	1 lobster = 1½ lb	1	136
boiled, poached, steamed	3 oz	1	83
	1 c	2	142
mussels, blue			
raw	3 oz	3	73
	1 c	6	129
boiled, poached, steamed	3 oz	6	147
octopus, common, raw	3 oz	2	70
oysters			
eastern			
raw	6 medium (70/qt)	3	58
	1 c	10	170
boiled, poached, steamed	6 medium (70/qt)	3	58
	3 oz	7	117
breaded & fried	3 oz	10	167
	6 medium (70/qt)	10	173
canned, solids & liquids	3 oz	3	58
	1 c	10	170
Pacific, raw	1 medium (20/qt)	2	41
	3 oz	4	69
scallops, mixed species			
raw	2 large (30/lb) or 5 small (75/lb)	1	26
	3 oz	2	75
breaded & fried	2 large (30/lb)	3	67
shrimp, mixed species			
raw	4 large (32/lb)	tr	30
	3 oz	1	90
boiled, poached, steamed	4 large (32/lb)	0	22
	3 oz	0	84
breaded & fried	4 large (32/lb)	4	73
	3 oz	10	206
canned, dry pack or drained	3 oz	1	102
solids of wet pack	1 c	1	154

	Portion	Carbohydrates (g)	Total Calories
snail, sea *See* whelk, *below*			
spiny lobster, mixed species,	3 oz	2	95
raw	1 lobster = 2 lb	5	233
squid, mixed species			
raw	3 oz	3	78
fried	3 oz	7	149
whelk			
raw	3 oz	7	117
boiled, poached, steamed	3 oz	13	233

Seafood Products

	Portion	Carbohydrates (g)	Total Calories
caviar, black & red, granular	1 T	1	40
	1 oz	1	71
crab cakes (blue crab)	2.1 oz	tr	93
fish sticks (walleye pollock), frozen, reheated	1 oz	7	76
gefilte fish, commercial, sweet recipe w/broth	1½ oz	3	35
imitation seafood, made from surimi			
crab, Alaska king	3 oz	9	87
scallops, mixed species	3 oz	9	84
shrimp, mixed species	3 oz	8	86
roe, mixed species, raw	1 oz	tr	39
surimi (processed from walleye pollock)	1 oz	2	28
	3 oz	6	84
tuna salad	3 oz	8	159
	1 c	19	383

▪ BRAND NAME

	Portion	Carbohydrates (g)	Total Calories
Featherweight			
salmon, pink	3⅞ oz	0	140
sardines			
canned in oil	1⅞ oz	0	109
canned in tomato	1⅞ oz	?	?
canned in water	1⅞ oz	0	109
tuna, light chunk	6½ oz	0	210
Fresh Chef			
seafood pasta salad	4¼ oz	15	240
Health Valley			
Best of Sea Food tuna	6½ oz	1	180
No Salt Diet tuna	6½ oz	0	200
Rokeach			
Natural Broth gefilte fish	1 ball = 2 oz	3	46

	Portion	Carbohydrates (g)	Total Calories
Old Vienna gefilte fish	1 ball = 2.6 oz	5	68
Old Vienna whitefish & pike gefilte fish	1 ball = 2.6 oz	5	70
whitefish & pike gefilte in jellied broth	1 ball = 2 oz	3	46

❑ SEASONINGS

See also BREADCRUMBS, CROUTONS, STUFFINGS, & SEASONED COATINGS; SAUCES, GRAVIES, & CONDIMENTS; VEGETABLES, PLAIN & PREPARED

NOTE: Most spices & herbs for which values are available contain fewer than 2 grams of carbohydrates & fewer than 10 calories per teaspoon. The following are exceptions.

cinnamon sugar	1 t	4	16
fenugreek seed	1 t	2	12
garlic powder	1 t	2	9
mustard seed, yellow	1 t	1	15
nutmeg	1 t	1	12
pepper, seasoned	1 t	2	10
poppy seed	1 t	1	15

▪ BRAND NAME

Featherweight

all salt substitutes	¼ t	0	0

Health Valley

all purpose	1 t	1	11
chicken	1 t	2	8
fish	1 t	2	11
steak/ham	1 t	1	6
vegetable	1 t	3	13

Kikkoman

teriyaki baste & glaze	1 t	2	9

Ortega

mild taco meat seasoning	1 oz	18	90

Shake 'n Bake Seasoning Mixture

Country Mild recipe	¼ pouch	10	80
Italian herb recipe	¼ pouch	15	80
Original Recipe			
for chicken	¼ pouch	14	80
for fish	¼ pouch	14	70
for pork	¼ pouch	16	80
for pork barbecue	¼ pouch	15	80

	Portion	Carbohydrates (g)	Total Calories

❏ **SEEDS & SEED-BASED BUTTERS, FLOURS, & MEALS**
See also NUTS & NUT-BASED BUTTERS, FLOURS, MEALS, MILKS, PASTES, & POWDERS

	Portion	Carbohydrates (g)	Total Calories
alfalfa seeds, sprouted, raw	1 c	1	10
breadfruit seeds			
raw	1 oz	8	54
boiled	1 oz	9	48
roasted	1 oz	11	59
breadnuttree seeds			
raw	1 oz	13	62
dried	1 oz	23	104
chia seeds, dried	1 oz	14	134
cottonseed flour			
partially defatted	1 T	2	18
	1 c	38	337
low-fat	1 oz	10	94
cottonseed kernels, roasted	1 T	2	51
	1 c	33	754
cottonseed meal, partially defatted	1 oz	11	104
lotus seeds			
raw	1 oz	5	25
dried	1 oz	18	94
	1 c	21	106
pumpkin & squash seeds			
whole, roasted	1 oz	15	127
	1 c	34	285
kernels			
dried	1 oz	5	154
	1 c	25	747
roasted	1 oz	4	148
	1 c	31	1,184
ramons *See* breadnuttree seeds, *above*			
safflower seed kernels, dried	1 oz	10	147
safflower seed meal, partially defatted	1 oz	14	97
sesame butter			
paste	1 oz	7	169
	1 T	4	95
tahini			
from raw & stone-ground kernels	1 oz	7	162
	1 T	4	86
from roasted & toasted kernels	1 oz	6	169
	1 T	3	89

	Portion	Carbohydrates (g)	Total Calories
sesame butter: tahini *(cont.)*			
from unroasted kernels	1 oz	5	173
	1 T	3	85
sesame flour			
high-fat	1 oz	8	149
partially defatted	1 oz	10	109
low-fat	1 oz	10	95
sesame meal, partially defatted	1 oz	7	161
sesame seeds			
whole			
dried	1 T	2	52
	1 c	34	825
roasted & toasted	1 oz	7	161
kernels			
dried	1 T	1	47
	1 c	14	882
toasted	1 oz	7	161
sisymbrium sp. seeds, whole,	1 oz	17	90
dried	1 c	43	235
squash seeds *See* pumpkin & squash seeds, *above*			
sunflower seed butter	1 T	4	93
sunflower seed flour, partially	1 T	2	16
defatted	1 c	29	261
sunflower seed kernels			
dried	1 oz	5	162
	1 c	27	821
dry roasted	1 oz	7	165
	1 c	31	745
oil roasted	1 oz	4	175
	1 c	20	830
toasted	1 oz	6	176
	1 c	28	829
tahini *See* sesame butter: tahini, *above*			
watermelon seed kernels, dried	1 oz	4	158
	1 c	17	602

- ## BRAND NAME

Arrowhead Mills

alfalfa seeds, sprouted	1 c	4	40
amaranth seeds	2 oz	35	200
flax seeds	1 oz	11	140
sesame seeds			
whole	1 oz	6	160
hulled	1 oz	4	160
sesame tahini, chemical-free	1 oz	4	170
sunflower seeds, hulled	1 oz	6	160

Planters

sunflower seeds	1 oz	5	160

	Portion	Carbohydrates (g)	Total Calories

❑ **SHERBETS** *See* DESSERTS, FROZEN

❑ **SHORTENINGS** *See* FATS, OILS, & SHORTENINGS

❑ **SNACKS**
See also CRACKERS

	Portion	Carbohydrates (g)	Total Calories
cheese puffs	1 oz	15	159
cheese straws	4	8	109
corn chips	1 oz	16	155
popcorn			
air-popped	1 c	6	30
popped in vegetable oil	1 c	6	55
sugar-syrup-coated	1 c	30	135
potato chips	10	10	105
made from dried potatoes	1 oz	12	164
potato sticks	1 oz	15	148
	½ c	10	94
pretzels			
stick	10	2	10
twisted, Dutch	1	13	65
twisted, thin	10	48	240
tortilla chips	1 oz	19	139

▪ **BRAND NAME**

Arrowhead Mills

	Portion	Carbohydrates (g)	Total Calories
popcorn, unpopped	2 oz	41	210
Cornnuts			
Original or unsalted	1 oz	19	120
barbecue or nacho cheese	1 oz	16	110
Del Monte			
pineapple nuggets	0.9 oz	22	90
Sierra trail mix	0.9 oz	13	130
tropical fruit mix	0.9 oz	20	90
yogurt raisins, plain or strawberry	0.9 oz	18	120
Featherweight			
cheese curls	1 oz	16	150
corn chips	1 oz	15	170
nacho cheese chips	1 oz	18	150
potato chips	1 oz	14	160
pretzels	3	4	20
round tortilla chips	1 oz	18	150

	Portion	Carbohydrates (g)	Total Calories
Health Valley			
CORN CHIPS			
corn chips, regular or no salt	1 oz	15	160
cheese corn chips			
regular	1 oz	13	160
no salt	1 oz	15	160
POTATO CHIPS			
Country Chips, regular or no salt	1 oz	14	160
Country Ripples, regular or no salt	1 oz	14	160
potato chips, regular or no salt	1 oz	14	160
potato chips, dip, regular or no salt	1 oz	14	160
SNACK PUFFS			
Carrot Lites	17	6	70
Cheddar Lites, regular, no salt, or w/green onion	17	4	40
TORTILLA CHIPS			
Buenitos: regular, no salt, or nacho cheese & chili	1 oz	17	150
Mister Salty Pretzels			
butter-flavored sticks	90	22	110
Dutch	2	22	110
Junior	29	22	110
Mini Mix	23	23	110
sticks	90	22	110
Veri-Thin sticks	45	22	110
Nabisco			
DOO DADS			
Original	1 oz or ½ c	18	140
cheddar & herb	1 oz or ½ c	18	140
Zesty cheese	1 oz or ½ c	18	140
GREAT CRISPS!			
cheese & chive	9	8	70
French onion	7	8	70
Italian	9	8	70
nacho	8	8	70
Real bacon	9	8	70
savory garlic	8	9	70
sesame	9	8	70
sour cream & onion	8	8	70
tomato & celery	9	8	70

	Portion	Carbohydrates (g)	Total Calories
NIPS			
Real cheddar cheese	13	9	70
pizza	20	9	70
taco	14	8	70
Pepperidge Farm			
SNACK STICKS			
Original	8	19	130
cheese or sesame	8	18	130
TINY GOLDFISH			
Original or cheddar cheese	45	18	140
Planters			
Cheez Balls	1 oz	14	160
Cheez Curls	1 oz	14	160
corn chips	1 oz	15	160
Fruit 'n Nut Mix	1 oz	13	150
popcorn	3 c popped	5	20
microwave, butter	3 c popped	13	140
microwave, natural	3 c popped	14	140
Potato Crunchies	1¼ oz	21	190
pretzels	1 oz	22	110
round toast crackers	4	15	140
sour cream & onion puffs	1 oz	16	160
square cheese crackers	4	15	140
Rokeach			
Dutch pretzels	1 oz	24	110

❑ SOUPS, PREPARED

Canned

	Portion	Carbohydrates (g)	Total Calories
asparagus, cream of, con- densed	1 can = 10¾ oz	26	210
prepared w/water	1 c	11	87
prepared w/whole milk	1 c	16	161
	1 can	40	392
bean, black, condensed	1 can = 11 oz	48	285
prepared w/water	1 c	20	116
bean w/bacon, condensed	1 can = 11½ oz	55	420
prepared w/water	1 c	23	173
bean w/frankfurter, condensed	1 can = 11¼ oz	53	454
prepared w/water	1 c	22	187
bean w/ham, chunky, ready-to- serve	1 c	27	231
	1 can = 19¼ oz	61	519

	Portion	Carbohydrates (g)	Total Calories
beef, chunky, ready-to-serve	1 c	20	171
	1 can = 19 oz	44	383
beef broth or bouillon, ready-	1 c	tr	16
to-serve	1 can = 14 oz	tr	27
beef mushroom, condensed	1 can = 10¾ oz	?	?
prepared w/water	1 c	?	?
beef noodle, condensed	1 can = 10¾ oz	22	204
prepared w/water	1 c	9	84
celery, cream of, condensed	1 can = 10¾ oz	21	219
prepared w/water	1 c	9	90
prepared w/whole milk	1 c	15	165
	1 can	35	400
cheese, condensed	1 can = 11 oz	26	377
prepared w/water	1 c	11	155
prepared w/whole milk	1 c	16	230
	1 can	39	558
chicken, chunky, ready-to-serve	1 c	17	178
	1 can = 10¾ oz	21	216
chicken, cream of, condensed	1 can = 10¾ oz	23	283
prepared w/water	1 c	9	116
prepared w/whole milk	1 c	15	191
	1 can	36	464
chicken & dumplings, condensed	1 can = 10½ oz	15	236
prepared w/water	1 c	6	97
chicken broth, condensed	1 can = 10¾ oz	2	94
prepared w/water	1 c	1	39
chicken gumbo, condensed	1 can = 10¾ oz	20	137
prepared w/water	1 c	8	56
chicken mushroom, condensed	1 can = 10¾ oz	?	?
prepared w/water	1 c	9	?
chicken noodle			
chunky, ready-to-serve	1 c	?	?
	1 can = 19 oz	?	?
condensed	1 can = 10½ oz	23	182
prepared w/water	1 c	9	75
chicken noodle w/meatballs,	1 c	8	99
ready-to-serve	1 can = 20 oz	19	227
chicken rice			
chunky, ready-to-serve	1 c	13	127
	1 can = 19 oz	29	286

	Portion	Carbohydrates (g)	Total Calories
condensed	1 can = 10½ oz	17	146
prepared w/water	1 c	7	60
chicken vegetable			
chunky, ready-to-serve	1 c	19	167
	1 can = 19 oz	42	374
condensed	1 can = 10½ oz	21	181
prepared w/water	1 c	9	74
chili beef, condensed	1 can = 11¼ oz	52	411
prepared w/water	1 c	21	169
clam chowder (Manhattan)			
chunky, ready-to-serve	1 c	19	133
	1 can = 19 oz	42	299
condensed	1 can = 10¾ oz	30	187
prepared w/water	1 c	12	78
clam chowder (New England), condensed	1 can = 10¾ oz	27	214
prepared w/water	1 c	12	95
prepared w/whole milk	1 c	17	163
	1 can	40	396
consommé w/gelatin, condensed	1 can = 10½ oz	4	71
prepared w/water	1 c	2	29
crab, ready-to-serve	1 c	10	76
	1 can = 13 oz	16	114
escarole, ready-to-serve	1 c	2	27
	1 can = 19½ oz	4	61
gazpacho, ready-to-serve	1 c	1	57
	1 can = 13 oz	1	87
lentil w/ham, ready-to-serve	1 c	20	140
	1 can = 20 oz	46	320
minestrone			
chunky, ready-to-serve	1 c	21	127
	1 can = 19 oz	47	285
condensed	1 can = 10½ oz	27	202
prepared w/water	1 c	11	83
mushroom, cream of, condensed	1 can = 10¾ oz	23	313
prepared w/water	1 c	9	129
prepared w/whole milk	1 c	15	203
	1 can	36	494
mushroom barley, condensed	1 can = 10¾ oz	?	?
prepared w/water	1 c	?	?

	Portion	Carbohydrates (g)	Total Calories
mushroom w/beef stock, condensed	1 can = 10¾ oz	23	208
prepared w/water	1 c	9	85
onion, condensed	1 can = 10½ oz	20	138
prepared w/water	1 c	8	57
onion, cream of, condensed	1 can = 10¾ oz	?	?
prepared w/water	1 c	?	?
oyster stew, condensed	1 can = 10½ oz	10	144
prepared w/water	1 c	4	59
prepared w/whole milk	1 c	10	134
	1 can	24	325
pea, green, condensed	1 can = 11¼ oz	64	398
prepared w/water	1 c	27	164
prepared w/whole milk	1 c	32	239
	1 can	78	579
pea, split, w/ham			
chunky, ready-to-serve	1 c	27	184
	1 can = 19 oz	60	413
condensed	1 can = 11½ oz	68	459
prepared w/water	1 c	28	189
pepperpot, condensed	1 can = 10½ oz	23	251
prepared w/water	1 c	9	103
potato, cream of, condensed	1 can = 10¾ oz	28	178
prepared w/water	1 c	11	73
prepared w/whole milk	1 c	17	148
	1 can	42	360
Scotch broth, condensed	1 can = 10½ oz	23	195
prepared w/water	1 c	9	80
shrimp, cream of, condensed	1 can = 10¾ oz	20	219
prepared w/water	1 c	8	90
prepared w/whole milk	1 c	14	165
	1 can	34	400
stockpot, condensed	1 can = 11 oz	28	242
prepared w/water	1 c	12	100
tomato, condensed	1 can = 10¾ oz	40	208
prepared w/water	1 c	17	86
prepared w/whole milk	1 c	22	160
	1 can	54	389
tomato beef w/noodle, condensed	1 can = 10¾ oz	51	341
prepared w/water	1 c	21	140

	Portion	Carbohydrates (g)	Total Calories
tomato bisque, condensed	1 can = 11 oz	58	300
prepared w/water	1 c	24	123
prepared w/whole milk	1 c	186	198
	1 can	452	481
tomato rice, condensed	1 can = 11 oz	53	291
prepared w/water	1 c	22	120
turkey, chunky, ready-to-serve	1 c	14	136
	1 can = 18¾ oz	32	306
turkey noodle, condensed	1 can = 10¾ oz	21	168
prepared w/water	1 c	9	69
turkey vegetable, condensed	1 can = 10½ oz	21	179
prepared w/water	1 c	9	74
vegetable, chunky, ready-to-serve	1 c	19	122
	1 can = 19 oz	43	274
vegetable, vegetarian, condensed	1 can = 10½ oz	29	176
prepared w/water	1 c	12	72
vegetable w/beef, condensed	1 can = 10¾ oz	25	192
prepared w/water	1 c	10	79
vegetable w/beef broth, condensed	1 can = 10½ oz	32	197
prepared w/water	1 c	13	81

Dehydrated

	Portion	Carbohydrates (g)	Total Calories
asparagus, cream of, prepared w/water	1 c	9	59
	39.7 oz	40	265
bean w/bacon, prepared w/water	1 c	16	105
beef broth or bouillon cubed	1 cube = 0.1 oz	1	6
prepared w/water	1 c	2	19
	6 fl oz	1	14
beef noodle, prepared w/water	1 c	6	41
	6 fl oz	4	30
cauliflower, prepared w/water	1 c	11	68
celery, cream of, prepared w/water	1 c	10	63
chicken, cream of, prepared w/water	1 c	13	107
	6 fl oz	10	80
chicken broth or bouillon cubed	1 cube = 0.2 oz	1	9
prepared w/water	1 c	1	21
	6 fl oz	1	16

	Portion	Carbohydrates (g)	Total Calories
chicken noodle	1 pkt = 2.6 oz	36	257
	1 pkt = 0.4 oz	5	38
prepared w/water	1 c	7	53
chicken rice, prepared w/water	1 c	9	60
chicken vegetable, prepared w/ water	1 c	8	49
	6 fl oz	6	37
clam chowder (Manhattan)	1 c	11	65
clam chowder (New England)	1 c	13	95
consommé, w/gelatin added, prepared w/water	1 c	2	17
	39½ oz	9	77
leek, prepared w/water	1 c	11	71
	36 fl oz	51	319
minestrone, prepared w/water	1 c	12	79
	40.2 oz	54	358
mushroom	1 pkt regular = 2.6 oz	38	328
	1 pkt instant = 0.6 oz	9	74
prepared w/water	1 c	11	96
onion	1 pkt = 1.4 oz	21	115
	1 pkt = ¼ oz	4	21
prepared w/water	1 c	5	28
oxtail, prepared w/water	1 c	9	71
	36 fl oz	40	318
pea, green or split	1 pkt = 4 oz	69	402
	1 pkt = 1 oz	17	100
prepared w/water	1 c	23	133
tomato (includes cream of tomato)	1 pkt = ¾ oz	15	77
prepared w/water	1 c	19	102
	6 fl oz	15	77
tomato vegetable (includes Italian vegetable & spring vegetable)	1 pkt = 1.4 oz	23	125
prepared w/water	1 c	10	55
	6 fl oz	8	41
vegetable, cream of, prepared w/water	1 c	12	105
	6 fl oz	9	79
vegetable beef, prepared w/ water	1 c	8	53
	1 pkt = 40 oz	36	240

• BRAND NAME

Campbell
CHUNKY SOUPS, READY-TO-SERVE

bean w/ham, Old Fashioned	11 oz	37	290
	9⅝ oz	33	260

	Portion	Carbohydrates (g)	Total Calories
beef	10¾ oz	23	190
	9½ oz	21	170
chicken, Old Fashioned	9½ oz	18	150
chicken mushroom, creamy	10½ oz	11	320
	9⅜ oz	10	280
chicken noodle	9½ oz	18	180
chicken noodle w/mushroom	10¾ oz	20	200
chicken rice	9½ oz	15	140
chicken vegetable	9½ oz	19	170
chili beef	11 oz	37	290
	9¾ oz	33	260
clam chowder (Manhattan style)	10¾ oz	24	160
	9½ oz	22	150
clam chowder (New England style)	10¾ oz	25	290
	9½ oz	22	250
Fisherman chowder	10¾ oz	26	260
	9½ oz	23	230
minestrone	9½ oz	26	160
mushroom, creamy	10½ oz	11	260
	9⅜ oz	10	240
sirloin burger	10¾ oz	23	220
	9½ oz	21	200
split pea & ham	10¾ oz	33	230
	9½ oz	29	210
steak & potato	10¾ oz	24	200
	9½ oz	21	170
Stroganoff-style beef	10¾ oz	28	300
turkey vegetable	9⅜ oz	16	150
vegetable	10¾ oz	23	140
	9½ oz	21	130
vegetable, Mediterranean	9½ oz	24	160
CONDENSED SOUPS, AS PACKAGED			
asparagus, cream of	4 oz	11	90
bean w/bacon	4 oz	21	150
beef broth (bouillon)	4 oz	1	16
beef noodle	4 oz	7	70
black bean	4 oz	17	110
celery, cream of	4 oz	8	100
cheddar cheese	4 oz	10	130
chicken, cream of	4 oz	9	110
chicken & dumplings	4 oz	9	80
chicken broth	4 oz	3	35
chicken gumbo	4 oz	8	60
chicken noodle	4 oz	8	70
chicken vegetable	4 oz	8	70

	Portion	Carbohydrates (g)	Total Calories
chicken w/rice	4 oz	7	60
chili beef	4 oz	17	130
clam chowder (Manhattan style)	4 oz	11	70
clam chowder (New England style)	4 oz	11	80
prepared w/whole milk	4 oz	17	150
French onion	4 oz	9	60
green pea	4 oz	25	160
minestrone	4 oz	14	80
mushroom, cream of	4 oz	9	100
mushroom, Golden	4 oz	10	80
nacho cheese	4 oz	5	100
noodles & ground beef	4 oz	10	90
onion, cream of	4 oz	12	100
prepared w/whole milk	4 oz	15	140
oyster stew	4 oz	5	80
prepared w/whole milk	4 oz	10	150
pepper pot	4 oz	9	90
potato, cream of	4 oz	11	70
prepared w/whole milk	4 oz	14	110
Scotch broth	4 oz	9	80
shrimp, cream of	4 oz	8	90
prepared w/whole milk	4 oz	13	160
Spanish-style vegetable (gazpacho)	4 oz	10	45
split pea w/ham & bacon	4 oz	24	160
tomato	4 oz	17	90
prepared w/whole milk	4 oz	22	160
tomato bisque	4 oz	23	120
tomato rice, Old Fashioned	4 oz	22	110
turkey noodle	4 oz	8	70
turkey vegetable	4 oz	8	70
vegetable	4 oz	14	90
vegetable, Old Fashioned	4 oz	9	60
vegetable, vegetarian	4 oz	15	90
vegetable beef	4 oz	10	70
won ton	4 oz	5	40

CREAMY NATURAL SOUPS, CONDENSED

asparagus, prepared w/whole milk	4 oz	18	170
potato, prepared w/whole milk	4 oz	17	190

DRY SOUP MIXES, AS PACKAGED

cheddar cheese	1 oz	12	160
chicken noodle	1 oz	15	100
chicken rice	1 oz	17	90
noodle	1 oz	19	110

	Portion	Carbohydrates (g)	Total Calories
onion	½ oz	10	50
onion mushroom	½ oz	10	50

HOME COOKIN' SOUPS, READY-TO-SERVE

chicken w/noodles	10¾ oz	12	140
country vegetable	10¾ oz	21	120
lentil	10¾ oz	29	170
minestrone	10¾ oz	22	140
split pea w/ham	10¾ oz	29	210
vegetable beef	10¾ oz	16	150

LOW-SODIUM SOUPS, READY-TO-SERVE

beef & mushroom, chunky	10¾ oz	23	210
chicken broth	10½ oz	2	40
chicken vegetable, chunky	10¾ oz	20	240
chicken w/noodles	10¾ oz	15	160
French onion	10½ oz	8	80
mushroom, cream of	10½ oz	17	200
split pea	10¾ oz	38	240
tomato w/tomato pieces	10½ oz	29	180
vegetable beef, chunky	10¾ oz	19	170

SEMICONDENSED SOUPS, AS PREPARED

bean w/ham, Old Fashioned	11 oz	30	220
chicken & noodles, Golden	11 oz	14	120
clam chowder (New England)	11 oz	19	130
prepared w/whole milk	11 oz	23	190
mushroom, savory cream of	11 oz	14	180
Tomato Royale	11 oz	35	180
vegetable, Old World	11 oz	18	130
vegetable beef & bacon, Burly	11 oz	20	160

College Inn
beef broth	1 c	1	18
chicken broth	1 c	0	35

Featherweight
bouillon, instant, beef or chicken	1 t	2	18
chicken noodle	3¾ oz	8	60
mushroom	3¾ oz	9	50
tomato	3¾ oz	13	60
vegetable beef	3¾ oz	12	80

Health Valley
bean, regular or no salt	4 oz	16	115
beef broth, regular or no salt	4 oz	2	10
chicken broth, regular or no salt	4 oz	1	30
clam chowder, regular or no salt	4 oz	8	80

	Portion	Carbohydrates (g)	Total Calories
green split pea			
regular	4 oz	14	70
no salt	4 oz	13	80
lentil, regular or no salt	4 oz	6	80
minestrone, regular or no salt	4 oz	10	90
minestrone, chunky, regular or no salt	4 oz	12	70
mushroom, regular or no salt	4 oz	8	70
potato, regular or no salt	4 oz	10	70
tomato, regular or no salt	4 oz	8	60
vegetable, regular or no salt	4 oz	9	80
vegetable, chunky, regular or no salt	4 oz	10	70
vegetable chicken, chunky, regular or no salt	4 oz	10	120
Nissin			
CUP O'NOODLES			
beef	1 pkg = 1 c	33	290
chicken	1 pkg = 1 c	32	300
shrimp	1 pkg = 1 c	32	300
HEARTY CUP O'NOODLES			
cream of chicken	1 pkg = 1 c	37	330
OODLES OF NOODLES			
beef	1 pkg = 1 c	49	390
chicken	1 pkg = 1 c	48	400
QUICK 'N TENDER			
chicken	1 pkg = 1 c	69	600
STIR 'N READY			
chicken	1 pkg = 1 c	21	190
TWIN CUP O'NOODLES			
chicken	1 pkg = 1 c	19	150
Rokeach			
CONDENSED SOUPS			
celery, cream of	5 oz	12	90
mushroom, cream of	5 oz	3	150
tomato	5 oz	20	90
tomato w/rice	5 oz	25	160
vegetarian vegetable	5 oz	15	90
READY-TO-SERVE SOUPS			
borscht	8 fl oz	22	96
Stouffer's Frozen Soups			
clam chowder (New England)	8 oz	16	200
spinach, cream of	8 oz	16	220
split pea w/ham	8¼ oz	30	200

	Portion	Carbohydrates (g)	Total Calories
Swanson			
beef broth	7¼ oz	1	20
chicken broth	7¼ oz	2	30

❑ SOUR CREAM *See* MILK, MILK SUBSTITUTES, & MILK PRODUCTS

❑ SOYBEANS & SOYBEAN PRODUCTS

Soybeans

boiled	½ c	9	149
dry roasted	½ c	28	387
mature seeds, sprouted			
raw	½ c	4	45
steamed	½ c	3	38
stir-fried	3½ oz	9	125
roasted	½ c	29	405

Soybean Products

fermented products			
miso	½ c	39	284
natto	½ c	13	187
tempeh	½ c	14	165
soy flour			
full-fat			
raw	½ c stirred	13	182
roasted	½ c stirred	13	184
low-fat	½ c stirred	15	163
defatted	½ c stirred	17	164
soy meal, defatted, raw	½ c	22	206
soy milk, fluid	1 c	4	79
soy protein			
concentrate	1 oz	7	92
isolate	1 oz	0	94
soy sauce			
made from hydrolyzed vegetable protein	1 T	1	7
	¼ c	4	24
made from soy (tamari)	1 T	1	11
	¼ c	3	35
made from soy & wheat (shoyu)	1 T	2	9
	¼ c	5	30
teriyaki sauce			
dehydrated	1 pkt = 1.6 oz	28	130
prepared w/water	1 c	28	131

	Portion	Carbohydrates (g)	Total Calories
teriyaki sauce *(cont.)*			
ready-to-serve	1 T	3	15
	1 fl oz	6	30
tofu			
raw			
regular	4.1 oz	2	88
	½ c	2	94
firm	2.9 oz	3	118
	½ c	5	183
dried-frozen (koyadofu)	0.6 oz	2	82
fried	½ oz	1	35
okara	½ c	8	47
salted & fermented (fuyu)	0.4 oz	1	13

▪ BRAND NAME

Arrowhead Mills
soybean flakes	2 oz	18	250
soybeans	2 oz	19	230
soy flour	2 oz	18	250
tamari soy sauce	1 T	2	15

Chun King
soy sauce	1 t	1	6

Fearn
lecithin granules	2 level T	2	100
liquid lecithin			
regular	1 T	0	130
mint-flavored	1 T	1	113
natural soya powder	¼ c	7	100
soya granules	¼ c	13	140
soya protein isolate	¼ c	0	60

Health Valley
Soy Moo soybean milk	8 fl oz	11	140
Tofu-Ya			
hard	4 oz	5	110
soft	4 oz	2	60

Kikkoman
soy sauce, regular or lite	1 T	1	10
stir-fry sauce	1 t	2	6
sweet & sour sauce	1 T	4	18
teriyaki sauce	1 T	3	15

❑ SPICES *See* SEASONINGS

	Portion	Carbohydrates (g)	Total Calories

❑ **STUFFINGS** *See* BREADCRUMBS, CROUTONS, STUFFINGS, & SEASONED COATINGS

❑ **SUGARS & SWEETENERS: HONEY, MOLASSES, SUGAR, SUGAR SUBSTITUTES, SYRUP, & TREACLE**

HONEY

	Portion	Carbohydrates (g)	Total Calories
honey	1 T	17	61
	5 T	78	306
MOLASSES			
first extraction, light	1 T	13	50
	5 T	65	252
second extraction, medium	1 T	12	46
	5 T	60	232
third extraction, blackstrap	1 T	11	43
	5 T	55	213
SUGAR			
brown	1 T	13	52
	5 T	94	364
maple	1 T	14	52
sugarcane juice	1 T	4	16
white			
granulated	1 cube	6	24
	1 t	4	16
	1 T	12	46
	½ c	100	385
powdered	1 T	11	42
	9 T	100	385
SYRUP			
cane	1 T	14	53
	5 T	68	263
corn	1 T	15	57
	5 T	74	287
dark corn	1 T	15	60
maple	1 T	13	50
	5 T	65	252
maple, imitation	1 T	15	55
	5 T	73	275
sorghum, pancake	1 T	13	52
table blend, pancake			
cane & maple	1 T	13	50

	Portion	Carbohydrates (g)	Total Calories
table blend, pancake *(cont.)*			
mainly corn	1 T	15	57
	5 T	74	286
TREACLE			
black	1 T	13	53
	5 T	67	265

● BRAND NAME

	Portion	Carbohydrates (g)	Total Calories
Aunt Jemima			
syrup	1 fl oz	26	103
Butter Lite syrup	1 fl oz	13	52
Lite syrup	1 fl oz	15	60
Brer Rabbit			
molasses, light or dark	1 T	14	60
Diamond Crystal			
sugar substitute	1 pkg	tr	1
Equal			
sugar substitute	1 pkg	1	4
Golden Griddle			
syrup	1 T	14	50
Grandma's Molasses			
gold label	1 T	17	70
green label	1 T	16	70
Karo			
corn syrup, dark or light	1 T	15	60
pancake syrup	1 T	15	60
Log Cabin			
syrup	1 fl oz	28	104
buttered syrup	1 fl oz	26	105
Country Kitchen syrup	1 fl oz	26	101
maple honey syrup	1 fl oz	28	106
NutraSweet			
sugar substitute	1 pkg	1	4
Sprinkle Sweet			
sugar substitute	1/8 t	1	2
Sugartwin			
sugar substitute			
white	1 pkg	1	3
white/brown	1 t	tr	1
Sweet & Low			
sugar substitute	1 pkg	1	4
Sweet 10			
sugar substitute	1/8 t	0	0
Vermont Maid			
syrup	1 T	13	50

	Portion	Carbohydrates (g)	Total Calories

❑ **SYRUP** *See* SUGARS & SWEETENERS

❑ **SYRUP, DESSERT** *See* DESSERT SAUCES, SYRUPS, & TOPPINGS

❑ **TOFU, FROZEN** *See* DESSERTS, FROZEN

❑ **TREACLE** *See* SUGARS & SWEETENERS

❑ **TURKEY** *See* POULTRY, FRESH & PROCESSED; PROCESSED MEAT & POULTRY PRODUCTS

❑ **VEAL** *See* LAMB, VEAL, & MISCELLANEOUS MEATS

❑ **VEGETABLES, PLAIN & PREPARED**
See also LEGUMES & LEGUME PRODUCTS; PICKLES, OLIVES, RELISHES, & CHUTNEYS; RICE & GRAINS, PLAIN & PREPARED

Vegetables, Plain

	Portion	Carbohydrates (g)	Total Calories
alfalfa seeds *See* SEEDS & SEED-BASED BUTTERS, FLOURS, & MEALS			
amaranth			
raw	1 c	1	7
boiled, drained	½ c	3	14
arrowhead			
raw	1 medium corm = 0.4 oz	2	12
boiled, drained	1 medium corm = 1.4 oz	2	9
artichokes, globe & French varieties			
boiled	1 medium = 4.2 oz	12	53
	½ c hearts	9	37
frozen, boiled, drained	9 oz pkg	22	108

	Portion	Carbohydrates (g)	Total Calories
artichokes, Jerusalem *See* Jerusalem artichokes, *below*			
asparagus, cuts & spears			
raw	4 spears = 2 oz	2	13
boiled	4 spears = 2.1 oz	3	15
canned			
drained solids	½ c	3	24
solids & liquids	½ c	3	17
frozen, boiled, drained	10 oz pkg	14	82
	4 spears = 2.1 oz	3	17
asparagus beans *See* yardlong beans, *under* LEGUMES & LEGUME PRODUCTS			
balsam pear			
leafy tips			
raw	½ c	1	7
boiled, drained	½ c	2	10
pods			
raw	1 c	3	16
boiled, drained	½ c	2	12
bamboo shoots			
raw	½ c	4	21
boiled, drained	1 c	2	15
canned, drained solids	1 c	4	25
basella *See* vinespinach, *below*			
beans, shellie, canned, solids & liquids	½ c	8	37
beans, snap			
raw	½ c	4	17
boiled, drained	½ c	5	22
canned			
drained solids	½ c	3	13
solids & liquids	½ c	4	18
solids & liquids, seasoned	½ c	4	18
frozen, boiled, drained	½ c	4	18
beet greens			
raw	½ c	1	4
boiled, drained	½ c	4	20
beets			
raw	½ c sliced	7	30
boiled, drained	½ c sliced	6	26
canned			
drained solids	½ c sliced	6	27
solids & liquids	½ c sliced	8	36
pickled, canned, solids & liquids	½ c	19	75
beets, Harvard, canned, solids & liquids	½ c	22	89
bittergourd; bittermelon *See* balsam pear, *above*			

	Portion	Carbohydrates (g)	Total Calories
bok choy *See* cabbage, Chinese, *below*			
borage			
raw	½ c	1	9
boiled, drained	3½ oz	4	25
broad beans *See* LEGUMES & LEGUME PRODUCTS			
broccoli			
raw	1 spear = 5.3 oz	8	42
boiled, drained	½ c	4	23
	1 spear = 6.3 oz	10	53
frozen, boiled, drained	½ c chopped	4	25
	½ c spears	13	69
	10 oz pkg spears	5	25
brussels sprouts			
boiled, drained	1 sprout = 0.73 oz	2	8
	½ c	7	30
frozen, boiled, drained	½ c	5	33
burdock root			
raw	1 c	20	85
	5½ oz	27	112
boiled, drained	1 c	26	110
	5.8 oz	35	146
butterbur			
raw	1 c	3	13
boiled, drained	3½ oz	2	8
cabbage			
raw	½ c shredded	2	8
boiled, drained	½ c shredded	4	16
cabbage, Chinese			
bok choy			
raw	½ c shredded	1	5
boiled, drained	½ c shredded	2	10
pe-tsai			
raw	½ c shredded	1	6
boiled, drained	1 c shredded	3	16
cabbage, red			
raw	½ c shredded	2	10
boiled, drained	½ c shredded	3	16
cabbage, savoy			
raw	½ c shredded	2	10
boiled, drained	½ c shredded	4	18
cardoon, raw	½ c shredded	4	18
carrots			
raw	½ c shredded	6	24
	2½ oz	7	31
boiled, drained	½ c sliced	8	35
	1.6 oz	5	21

	Portion	Carbohydrates (g)	Total Calories
carrots *(cont.)*			
canned			
drained solids	½ c sliced	4	17
solids & liquids	½ c sliced	6	28
frozen, boiled, drained	½ c sliced	6	26
cassava, raw	3½ oz	27	120
cauliflower			
raw	½ c pieces	2	12
	3 flowerets = 2 oz	3	13
boiled, drained	½ c pieces	3	15
frozen, boiled, drained	½ c pieces	3	17
celeriac			
raw	½ c	7	31
boiled, drained	3½ oz	6	25
celery			
raw	1 stalk = 1.4 oz	1	6
	½ c diced	2	9
boiled, drained	½ c diced	3	11
celtuce, raw	1 leaf = 0.3 oz	tr	2
chard, Swiss			
raw	½ c chopped	1	3
boiled, drained	½ c chopped	4	18
chayote, fruit			
raw	1 c pieces	7	32
	7.1 oz	11	49
boiled, drained	1 c pieces	8	38
chicory, raw			
greens	½ c chopped	4	21
roots	½ c pieces	8	33
witloof	½ c	1	7
Chinese parsley *See* coriander, *below*			
Chinese preserving melon *See* wax gourd, *below*			
chives			
raw	1 t	tr	0
	1 T	tr	1
freeze-dried	1 T	tr	1
chrysanthemum, garland			
raw	1 c pieces	1	4
boiled, drained	½ c pieces	2	10
collards			
raw	½ c chopped	4	18
boiled, drained	½ c chopped	3	13
frozen, boiled, drained	½ c chopped	6	31
coriander (cilantro), raw	¼ c	tr	1
corn, sweet			
raw	½ c kernels	15	66
	kernels from 1 ear	17	77

	Portion	Carbohydrates (g)	Total Calories
boiled, drained	½ c kernels	21	89
	kernels from 1 ear	20	83
canned			
cream style	½ c	23	93
in brine, drained solids	½ c	15	66
in brine, solids & liquids	½ c	19	79
vacuum pack	½ c	20	83
w/red & green peppers, solids & liquids	½ c	21	86
frozen, boiled, drained	½ c kernels	17	67
	kernels from 1 ear	14	59
cowpeas *See* LEGUMES & LEGUME PRODUCTS			
cress, garden			
raw	1 sprig	tr	0
	½ c	1	8
boiled, drained	½ c	3	16
cucumber, raw	½ c sliced	2	7
	10½ oz	9	39
daikon *See* radishes: Oriental, *below*			
dandelion greens			
raw	½ c chopped	3	13
boiled, drained	½ c chopped	3	17
dasheen *See* taro, *below*			
dock			
raw	½ c chopped	2	15
boiled, drained	3½ oz	3	20
eggplant, boiled, drained	1 c cubed	6	27
endive, raw	½ c chopped	1	4
endive, Belgian *See* chicory: witloof, *above*			
eppaw, raw	½ c	16	75
escarole *See* endive, *above*			
garlic, raw	1 clove = 0.1 oz	1	4
ginger root, raw	0.4 oz	2	8
	¼ c sliced	4	17
gourd			
dishcloth, boiled, drained	½ c sliced	13	50
white-flowered (calabash), boiled, drained	½ c cubed	3	11
horseradish-tree			
leafy tips			
raw	½ c chopped	1	6
boiled, drained	½ c chopped	2	13
pods			
raw	1 pod = 0.4 oz	1	4
boiled, drained	½ c sliced	5	21
hyacinth beans *See* LEGUMES & LEGUME PRODUCTS			
Jerusalem artichokes, raw	½ c sliced	13	57

	Portion	Carbohydrates (g)	Total Calories
jicama *See* yam bean, *below*			
jute (pot herb), boiled, drained	½ c	3	16
kale			
raw	½ c chopped	3	17
boiled, drained	½ c chopped	4	21
frozen, boiled, drained	½ c chopped	3	20
kale, Scotch			
raw	½ c chopped	3	14
boiled, drained	½ c chopped	4	18
kanpyo (dried gourd strips)	0.7 oz	12	49
kohlrabi			
raw	½ c sliced	4	19
boiled, drained	½ c sliced	5	24
lamb's-quarters, boiled, drained	½ c chopped	5	29
leeks			
raw	¼ c chopped	4	16
boiled, drained	¼ c chopped	2	8
freeze-dried	1 T	tr	1
lentils *See* LEGUMES & LEGUME PRODUCTS			
lettuce, raw			
butterhead (includes Boston & Bibb types)	2 leaves = ½ oz	tr	2
	1 head = 5.7 oz	4	21
cos or romaine	1 inner leaf = 0.35 oz	tr	2
	½ c shredded	1	4
iceberg	1 leaf = 0.7 oz	tr	3
	1 head = 1 lb 3 oz	11	70
looseleaf	1 leaf = 0.35 oz	tr	2
	½ c shredded	1	5
lima beans *See* LEGUMES & LEGUME PRODUCTS			
lotus root, boiled, drained	3.1 oz	14	59
manioc *See* cassava, *above*			
mountain yam, Hawaii, steamed	½ c	14	59
mung beans *See* LEGUMES & LEGUME PRODUCTS			
mushrooms			
raw	½ c pieces	2	9
boiled, drained	½ c pieces	4	21
canned, drained solids	½ c pieces	4	19
mushrooms, shitake			
dried	0.1 oz	3	11
cooked	½ oz	10	40
mustard greens			
raw	½ c chopped	1	7
boiled, drained	½ c chopped	1	11
frozen, boiled, drained	½ c chopped	2	14

	Portion	Carbohydrates (g)	Total Calories
mustard spinach			
raw	½ c chopped	3	17
boiled, drained	½ c chopped	3	14
New Zealand spinach			
raw	½ c chopped	1	4
boiled, drained	½ c chopped	2	11
okra			
boiled, drained	½ c sliced	6	25
frozen, boiled, drained	½ c sliced	8	34
onions			
raw	1 T chopped	1	3
	½ c chopped	6	27
boiled, drained	1 T chopped	1	4
	½ c chopped	7	29
canned, solids & liquids	2.2 oz	3	12
dehydrated flakes	1 T	4	16
frozen, boiled, drained	1 T chopped	1	4
	½ c chopped	7	30
onions, spring, raw	1 T chopped	tr	2
	½ c chopped	3	13
onions, Welsh, raw	3½ oz	7	34
oysterplant See salsify, below			
parsley			
raw	10 sprigs = 0.35 oz	1	3
	½ c chopped	2	10
freeze-dried	1 T	tr	1
parsnips			
raw	½ c sliced	12	50
boiled, drained	½ c sliced	15	63
peas, edible pods			
raw	½ c	5	30
boiled, drained	½ c	6	34
frozen, boiled, drained	½ c	7	42
	10 oz pkg	23	132
peas, green			
raw	½ c	11	63
boiled, drained	½ c	13	67
canned			
drained solids	½ c	11	59
solids & liquids	½ c	11	61
solids & liquids, seasoned	½ c	11	57
frozen, boiled, drained	½ c	11	63
peas, mature seeds, sprouted			
raw	½ c	17	77
boiled, drained	3½ oz	22	118
peas, split See split peas, under LEGUMES & LEGUME PRODUCTS			
peas & carrots			
canned, solids & liquids	½ c	11	48
frozen, boiled, drained	½ c	8	38
	10 oz pkg	28	133

	Portion	Carbohydrates (g)	Total Calories
peas & onions			
canned, solids & liquids	½ c	5	30
frozen, boiled, drained	½ c	8	40
pepeao			
raw	0.2 oz	tr	2
dried	½ c	10	36
peppers			
hot chili			
raw	1 pepper = 1.6 oz	4	18
	½ c chopped	7	30
canned, solids & liquids	1 pepper = 2.6 oz	4	18
	½ c chopped	4	17
jalapeño, canned, solids & liquids	½ c chopped	3	17
sweet			
raw	1 pepper = 2.6 oz	4	18
	½ c chopped	3	12
boiled, drained	1 pepper = 2.6 oz	3	13
	½ c chopped	3	12
canned, solids & liquids	½ c halves	3	13
freeze-dried	1 T	tr	1
	¼ c	1	5
frozen, unprepared, chopped	10 oz pkg	13	58
frozen, boiled, drained	3½ oz chopped	4	18
pigeon peas See LEGUMES & LEGUME PRODUCTS			
pimientos See PICKLES, OLIVES, RELISHES, & CHUTNEYS			
pinto beans See LEGUMES & LEGUME PRODUCTS			
poi	½ c	33	134
pokeberry shoots			
raw	½ c	3	18
boiled, drained	½ c	3	16
potatoes			
raw			
flesh	3.9 oz	20	88
skin	1.3 oz	5	22
baked			
flesh & skin	7.1 oz	51	220
flesh	5½ oz	39	145
skin	2 oz	27	115
boiled in skin			
flesh	4.8 oz	27	119
skin	1.2 oz	6	27
boiled w/out skin, flesh	4.8 oz	27	116
canned			
drained solids	1.2 oz	5	21
solids & liquids	1 c	26	120

	Portion	Carbohydrates (g)	Total Calories
frozen, whole, unprepared	½ c	16	71
microwaved in skin			
flesh & skin	7.1 oz	49	212
flesh	5½ oz	36	156
skin	2 oz	17	77
pumpkin			
boiled, drained	½ c mashed	6	24
canned	½ c	10	41
pumpkin flowers			
raw	1 c	1	5
boiled, drained	½ c	2	10
pumpkin leaves, boiled, drained	½ c	1	7
purslane			
raw	1 c	1	7
boiled, drained	1 c	4	21
radishes, raw	10 radishes = 1.6 oz	2	7
Oriental			
raw	½ c	2	8
boiled, drained	½ c sliced	3	13
dried	½ c	37	157
white icicle, raw	½ c sliced	1	7
radish seeds, sprouted, raw	½ c	1	8
rutabagas			
raw	½ c cubed	6	25
boiled, drained	½ c cubed	7	29
	½ c mashed	9	41
salsify			
raw	½ c sliced	12	55
boiled, drained	½ c sliced	10	46
seaweed			
agar, raw	3½ oz	7	26
kelp, raw	3½ oz	10	43
laver, raw	3½ oz	5	35
spirulina			
raw	3½ oz	2	26
dried	3½ oz	24	290
wakame, raw	3½ oz	9	45
sesbania flower			
raw	1 c	1	5
steamed	1 c	5	23
shallots			
raw	1 T chopped	2	7
freeze-dried	1 T	1	3
snow peas See peas, edible pods, *above*			
soybeans See SOYBEANS & SOYBEAN PRODUCTS			
spinach			
raw	½ c chopped	1	6
boiled, drained	½ c	3	21

	Portion	Carbohydrates (g)	Total Calories
spinach *(cont.)*			
canned			
drained solids	½ c	4	25
solids & liquids	½ c	3	22
frozen, boiled, drained	½ c	5	27
	10 oz pkg	12	63
spinach, mustard *See* mustard spinach, *above*			
spinach, New Zealand *See* New Zealand spinach, *above*			
sprouts *See plant name (alfalfa, mung bean, etc.)*			
squash, summer			
all varieties			
raw	½ c sliced	3	13
boiled, drained	½ c sliced	4	18
crookneck			
raw	½ c sliced	3	12
boiled, drained	½ c sliced	4	18
canned, drained solids	½ c sliced	3	14
frozen, boiled, drained	½ c sliced	5	24
scallop			
raw	½ c sliced	3	12
boiled, drained	½ c sliced	3	14
zucchini			
raw	½ c sliced	2	9
boiled, drained	½ c sliced	4	14
canned, Italian style, in tomato sauce	½ c	8	33
frozen, boiled, drained	½ c	4	19
squash, winter			
all varieties			
raw	½ c cubed	5	21
baked	½ c cubed	9	39
acorn			
baked	½ c cubed	15	57
boiled	½ c mashed	11	41
butternut			
baked	½ c cubed	11	41
frozen, boiled	½ c mashed	12	47
hubbard			
baked	½ c cubed	11	51
boiled	½ c mashed	8	35
spaghetti, boiled, drained, baked	½ c	5	23
string beans *See* beans, snap, *above*			
succotash			
boiled, drained	½ c	23	111
canned			
w/cream-style corn	½ c	23	102
w/whole kernel corn, solids & liquids	½ c	18	81
frozen, boiled, drained	½ c	17	79

	Portion	Carbohydrates (g)	Total Calories
swamp cabbage			
raw	1 c chopped	2	11
boiled, drained	1 c chopped	4	20
sweet potatoes			
baked in skin	½ c mashed	24	103
	1 potato = 4 oz	28	118
boiled w/out skin	½ c mashed	40	172
candied	3.7 oz	29	144
canned			
in syrup, drained solids	1 c	50	213
in syrup, solids & liquids	1 c	48	202
mashed	1 c	59	258
vacuum packed	1 c pieces	42	183
	1 c mashed	54	233
frozen, baked	½ c cubed	21	88
sweet potato leaves			
raw	1 c chopped	2	12
steamed	1 c	5	22
Swiss chard See chard, Swiss, above			
taro			
raw	½ c sliced	14	56
cooked	½ c sliced	23	94
taro chips	10 chips = 0.8 oz	16	110
taro leaves			
raw	1 c	2	12
steamed	1 c	6	35
taro shoots			
raw	1 shoot = 2.9 oz	2	9
cooked	½ c sliced	2	10
taro, Tahitian			
raw	½ c sliced	4	25
cooked	½ c sliced	5	30
tomatoes, green, raw	1 tomato = 4.3 oz	6	30
tomatoes, red, ripe			
raw	1 tomato = 4.3 oz	5	24
boiled	½ c	7	30
canned			
stewed	½ c	8	34
wedges in juice	½ c	8	34
w/green chilies	½ c	4	18
whole	½ c	5	24
stewed	1 c	10	59
tomato paste, canned	½ c	25	110
tomato puree, canned	1 c	25	102

tomato sauce See SAUCES, GRAVIES, & CONDIMENTS
towel gourd See gourd: dishcloth, above

	Portion	Carbohydrates (g)	Total Calories
tree fern, cooked	½ c chopped	8	28
turnip greens			
raw	½ c chopped	2	7
boiled, drained	½ c chopped	3	15
canned, solids & liquids	½ c	3	17
frozen, boiled, drained	½ c	4	24
turnip greens & turnips, frozen, boiled, drained	3½ oz	3	17
turnips			
raw	½ c cubed	4	18
boiled, drained	½ c cubed	4	14
frozen, boiled, drained	3½ oz	4	23
vegetables, mixed			
canned			
drained solids	½ c	8	39
solids & liquids	½ c	9	44
frozen, boiled, drained	½ c	12	54
	10 oz pkg	36	163
vinespinach, raw	3½ oz	3	19
water chestnuts, Chinese			
raw	1¼ oz	9	38
canned, solids & liquids	1 oz	3	14
watercress, raw	½ c chopped	tr	2
wax beans *See* beans, snap, *above*			
wax gourd (Chinese preserving melon), boiled, drained	½ c cubed	3	11
winged beans *See* LEGUMES & LEGUME PRODUCTS			
yam, baked or boiled	½ c cubed	19	79
yam bean (tuber only)			
raw	1 c sliced	11	49
boiled, drained	3½ oz	10	46
yardlong beans *See* LEGUMES & LEGUME PRODUCTS			
zucchini *See* squash, summer, *above*			

Vegetables, Prepared

coleslaw	½ c	7	42
corn pudding	1 c	32	271
onion rings, breaded, frozen, heated in oven	0.7 oz	8	81
potato chips & sticks *See* SNACKS			
potatoes, au gratin			
dry mix, prepared	5½ oz pkg	106	764
homemade	½ c	14	160
potatoes, french fried, frozen			
fried in animal fat & vegetable oil	1.8 oz	20	158
fried in vegetable oil	1.8 oz	20	158
heated in oven	1.8 oz	17	111
cottage-cut, heated in oven	1.8 oz	17	109
extruded, heated in oven	1.8 oz	19	163

	Portion	Carbohydrates (g)	Total Calories
potatoes, hashed brown			
frozen, plain, prepared	½ c	22	170
frozen, w/butter sauce, unprepared	6 oz pkg	31	229
homemade, prepared in vegetable oil	½ c	17	163
potatoes, mashed			
dehydrated flakes, prepared (whole milk & butter added)	½ c	16	118
granules w/milk, prepared	½ c	14	83
granules w/out milk, prepared (whole milk & butter added)	½ c	18	137
homemade w/whole milk & margarine	½ c	18	111
homemade w/whole milk	½ c	18	81
potatoes, O'Brien			
frozen, prepared	3½ oz	22	204
homemade	1 c	30	157
potatoes, scalloped			
dry mix, prepared w/whole milk & butter	5½ oz pkg	105	764
homemade	½ c	13	105
potato flour See FLOURS & CORNMEALS			
potato pancakes, homemade	2.7 oz	26	495
potato puffs, frozen, fried in vegetable oil	¼ oz	2	16
potato salad	½ c	14	179
sauerkraut, canned, solids & liquids	½ c	5	22
spinach soufflé	1 c	3	218

▪ BRAND NAME

	Portion	Carbohydrates (g)	Total Calories
Arrowhead Mills			
potato flakes	2 oz	44	140
B&B			
mushrooms, canned	2 oz	3	25
Birds Eye Frozen Vegetables *REGULAR*			
asparagus cuts	3.3 oz	4	25
beans			
baby lima	3.3 oz	24	130
cut or French cut green	3 oz	6	25
Italian green	3 oz	7	30
broccoli, chopped or cuts	3.3 oz	5	25
brussels sprouts	3.3 oz	7	35
cauliflower	3.3 oz	5	25

	Portion	Carbohydrates (g)	Total Calories
corn, sweet	3.3 oz	20	80
corn on the cob	1 ear	29	120
mixed vegetables	3.3 oz	13	60
onions, small whole	4 oz	10	40
peas, green	3.3 oz	13	80
spinach			
chopped	3.3 oz	3	20
whole leaf	3.3 oz	4	20
squash, cooked winter	4 oz	11	45

CHEESE SAUCE COMBINATIONS

baby brussels sprouts w/cheese sauce	4½ oz	12	110
broccoli w/cheese sauce	5 oz	12	120
broccoli w/creamy Italian cheese sauce	4½ oz	7	90
cauliflower w/cheese sauce	5 oz	12	110
peas & pearl onions w/cheese sauce	5 oz	18	140

COMBINATION

broccoli, carrots, pasta twists	3.3 oz	11	90
corn, green beans, pasta curls	3.3 oz	15	110
creamed spinach	3 oz	5	60
fresh green beans w/toasted almonds	3 oz	8	50
green peas & pearl onions	3.3 oz	13	70
green peas & potatoes w/cream sauce	2.6 oz	15	130
mixed vegetables w/onion sauce	2.6 oz	12	100
rice & green peas w/mushrooms	2.3 oz	23	110
small onions w/cream sauce	3 oz	11	110

DELUXE

artichoke hearts	3 oz	7	30
beans, whole green	3 oz	5	25
broccoli florets	3.3 oz	5	25
carrots, baby peas, & pearl onions	3.3 oz	10	50
carrots, whole baby	3.3 oz	9	40
corn, tender sweet	3.3 oz	20	80
peas, tender tiny	3.3 oz	11	60

FARM FRESH MIXTURES

broccoli, baby carrots, water chestnuts	3.2 oz	8	35
broccoli, cauliflower, carrots	3.2 oz	5	25
broccoli, corn, red peppers	3.2 oz	11	50

	Portion	Carbohydrates (g)	Total Calories
broccoli, green beans, pearl onions, red peppers	3.2 oz	5	25
broccoli, red peppers, bamboo shoots, straw mushrooms	3.2 oz	5	25
brussels sprouts, cauliflower, carrots	3.2 oz	7	30
cauliflower, baby whole carrots, snow pea pods	3.2 oz	6	30

INTERNATIONAL RECIPES

Bavarian style	3.3 oz	11	110
Chinese style	3.3 oz	8	80
chow mein style	3.3 oz	12	90
Italian style	3.3 oz	12	110
Japanese style	3.3 oz	10	100
Mandarin style	3.3 oz	12	90
New England style	3.3 oz	14	130
pasta primavera style	3.3 oz	14	120
San Francisco style	3.3 oz	11	100

STIR-FRY

Chinese style	3.3 oz	8	35
Japanese style	3.3 oz	7	30
Chun King			
bamboo shoots	2 oz	3	16
bean sprouts	4 oz	7	40
chow mein vegetables	4 oz	6	35
water chestnuts, whole, sliced	2 oz	10	45
Claussen			
sauerkraut	½ c	3	17
Fresh Chef			
Holiday cole slaw	4 oz	16	200
Old Fashioned potato salad	4 oz	19	210
Joan of Arc			
garden salad	½ c	17	80
potato salad			
German style	½ c	24	120
Home Style	½ c	19	160
pumpkin	½ c	11	50
sweet potatoes			
cut	½ c	25	110
in orange pineapple sauce	½ c	43	180
mashed	½ c	31	130
whole, packed in heavy syrup	½ c	35	150
wax beans, cut	½ c	5	25

	Portion	Carbohydrates (g)	Total Calories
Le Sueur			
CANNED			
asparagus spears	½ c	4	30
whole kernel corn	½ c	18	80
FROZEN, IN BUTTER SAUCE			
early peas	½ c	15	90
minipeas, pea pods, & water chestnuts	½ c	10	80
peas, carrots, & onions	½ c	11	80
Mexicorn			
Mexicorn w/peppers	½ c	18	80
Mrs. Paul's Prepared Vegetables			
candied yams	4 oz	48	200
corn fritters	2	33	250
eggplant parmigiana	5½ oz	20	270
fried eggplant sticks	3½ oz	29	240
onion rings, crispy	2½ oz	20	180
zucchini sticks, light batter	3 oz	21	200
Ortega			
green chiles, whole, diced, strips, sliced	1 oz	8	10
hot peppers, whole, diced	1 oz	2	8
jalapeño peppers, whole, diced	1 oz	3	10
tomatoes & jalapeños	1 oz	1	8
Pepperidge Farm Vegetables in Pastry			
broccoli w/cheese	1	18	250
cauliflower & cheese sauce	1	19	210
Pillsbury			
BUTTER SAUCE VEGETABLES			
baby lima beans	½ c	18	110
broccoli cauliflower carrots	½ c	4	30
broccoli spears	½ c	5	45
brussel sprouts	½ c	9	60
cauliflower	½ c	4	30
cut green beans	½ c	5	35
cut leaf spinach	½ c	6	60
French-style green beans	½ c	6	40
mixed vegetables	½ c	13	80
Niblets corn	½ c	18	100
sweet peas	½ c	14	90
CANNED VEGETABLES			
asparagus cuts	½ c	2	20
cream-style corn	½ c	21	100
cut green beans	½ c	3	20
Golden Shoe Peg corn	½ c	18	90
mushrooms	2 oz	2	14
mushrooms in butter sauce	2 oz	3	25

	Portion	Carbohydrates (g)	Total Calories
sweet peas	½ c	11	60
sweet peas & onions	½ c	11	60
three bean salad	½ c	18	80
whole kernel corn, vacuum pack	½ c	20	90

CREAM & CHEESE SAUCE COMBINATION

	Portion	Carbohydrates (g)	Total Calories
baby brussels sprouts in cheese-flavored sauce	½ c	13	80
broccoli cauliflower carrots in cheese-flavored sauce	½ c	9	70
broccoli in cheese-flavored sauce	½ c	9	70
broccoli in white cheddar cheese–flavored sauce	½ c	6	60
cauliflower in cheese-flavored sauce	½ c	10	60
cauliflower in white cheddar cheese–flavored sauce	½ c	7	70
creamed spinach	½ c	10	80
cream-style corn	½ c	25	120
peas in cream sauce	½ c	12	100

HARVEST FRESH

	Portion	Carbohydrates (g)	Total Calories
broccoli spears	½ c	4	30
cut broccoli	½ c	4	25
cut green beans	½ c	4	20
early June peas	½ c	13	80
lima beans	½ c	11	70
mixed vegetables	½ c	9	45
Niblets corn	½ c	18	90
spinach	½ c	5	40
sweet peas	½ c	12	60

HARVEST GET TOGETHERS

	Portion	Carbohydrates (g)	Total Calories
Broccoli Cauliflower Medley	½ c	10	60
Broccoli Fanfare	½ c	12	70
Cauliflower Carrot Bonanza	½ c	7	60

POLYBAG VEGETABLES

	Portion	Carbohydrates (g)	Total Calories
broccoli cuts	½ c	2	16
brussels sprouts	½ c	6	30
cauliflower cuts	½ c	2	12
green beans	½ c	4	20
lima beans	½ c	19	100
mixed vegetables	½ c	11	50
Niblets corn	½ c	17	80
Niblets corn on the cob	1 ear	32	150
sweet peas	½ c	11	60

	Portion	Carbohydrates (g)	Total Calories
POTATO SIDE DISHES			
stuffed baked potato w/cheese-flavored topping	1	33	200
stuffed baked potato w/sour cream & chives	1	31	230
VALLEY COMBINATION DUAL POUCH W/SAUCE			
American-style vegetables	½ c	16	90
Broccoli Cauliflower Medley	½ c	9	60
Broccoli Fanfare	½ c	13	80
Italian-style vegetables	½ c	5	50
Japanese-style vegetables	½ c	7	45
Le Sueur–style vegetables	½ c	13	90
Mexican-style vegetables	½ c	22	150
VALLEY COMBINATIONS, POLYBAG			
Broccoli Carrot Fanfare	½ c	4	20
Broccoli Cauliflower Supreme	½ c	3	18
Cauliflower Green Bean Festival	½ c	3	16
Corn Broccoli Bounty	½ c	8	45
Sweet Pea Cauliflower Medley	½ c	5	30
Stouffer			
broccoli in cheddar cheese sauce	4½ oz	7	150
corn soufflé	4 oz	16	150
creamed spinach	4½ oz	9	190
green bean mushroom casserole	4¾ oz	12	170
potatoes au gratin	⅓ of 11½ oz pkg	13	120
scalloped potatoes	4 oz	11	110
spinach soufflé	4 oz	10	140
yams & apples	5 oz	33	160
Vlasic			
Old Fashioned sauerkraut	1 oz	1	4

❏ **VINEGAR** *See* SALAD DRESSINGS, MAYONNAISE, VINEGAR, & DIPS

❏ **WHEY** *See* MILK, MILK SUBSTITUTES, & MILK PRODUCTS

	Portion	Carbohydrates (g)	Total Calories

❑ **YOGURT** *See* MILK, MILK SUBSTITUTES, & MILK PRODUCTS

❑ **YOGURT, FROZEN** *See* DESSERTS, FROZEN